1918 SPANISH FLU

———— ♦◇♦ ————

The Terrible Story of The Great Influenza, the 20th Century's Deadliest Pandemic

JOHN MUAN

Copyright @ by John Muan 2020 - All rights reserved.

This book is written with the sole purpose of providing relevant information on a specific topic for which every reasonable effort has been made to ensure that it is both accurate and reasonable. Nevertheless, by purchasing this book you consent to the fact that the author, as well as the publisher, are in no way experts on the topics contained herein, regardless of any claims as such that may be made within. As such, any suggestions or recommendations that are made within are done so purely for entertainment value. It is recommended that you always consult a professional, prior to undertaking any of the advice or techniques discussed within.

This is a legally binding declaration that is considered both valid and fair by both the Committee of Publishers Association and the American Bar Association and should be considered as legally binding within the United States.

The reproduction, transmission, and duplication of any of the content found herein, including any specific or extended information will be done as an illegal act regardless of the end form the information ultimately takes. This includes copied versions of the work both physical, digital and audio unless express consent of the Publisher is provided beforehand. Any additional rights reserved.

Furthermore, the information that can be found within the pages described forthwith shall be considered both accurate and truthful when it comes to the recounting of facts. As such, any use, correct or incorrect, of the provided information will render the Publisher free of responsibility as to the actions taken outside of their direct purview. Regardless, there are zero scenarios where the original author or the Publisher can be deemed liable in any fashion for any damages or hardships that may result from any of the information discussed herein.

Additionally, the information in the following pages is intended only for informational purposes and should thus be thought of as universal. As befitting its nature, it is presented without assurance regarding its prolonged validity or interim quality. Trademarks that are mentioned are done without written consent and can in no way be considered an endorsement from the trademark holder

Cover: "Members of the War Camp Community Committee make flu masks"- EPA

TABLE OF CONTENTS

INTRODUCTION 7

CHAPTER 1 - VIRUS' ANALYSIS 11
   What caused Spanish influenza? 12
   For what reason was it called the Spanish flu? 14
   What were the symptoms of the flu? 15
   Development 17

CHAPTER 2 - ORIGINS AND CAUSES 25
   Three Waves of Spanish Flu 25
      First Wave: Springtime in Spain, 1918 25
      Second Wave: Autumn and winter in Spain, 1918 ... 28
      Third Wave: Winter and spring in Spain, 1919 34
      What number of people died from Spanish flu? 42

CHAPTER 3 - CONSEQUENCES OF VIRUS 45
   Spanish influenza Orphans 45
   The Spanish flu in Kingston 68
   The search for a vaccine 73
   How the 1918 Flu Pandemic Helped Shape Respiratory Care 75
      Wakeup call 76
      The new spotlight on antibodies 77
      RTS are key players 78

CHAPTER 4 - SPANISH FLU TREATMENTS 85
   Antibody Development over the US 87
   Estimating Achievement 92
      Clinical Performances of the Day 94
      Skulls, skeletons, and stones 96
      The enigma of cultural amnesia 98
      Grief behind closed doors 99
      Deaths that defy imagination 101

CHAPTER 5 - BIOGRAPHICAL TESTIMONIES 103
   Young students bring overlooked stories of the Spanish flu back to life 103
      A deadly and largely forgotten enemy 105
      Amelia Earhart and the Spanish Flu in Canada 107
   Elizabeth "Kirkina" Jefferies Mucko and the effect on general wellbeing 108
      Honoring memories 109
   Survivors remember 1918 worldwide flu pandemic .. 110

CHAPTER 6 - WHAT WE CAN LEARN 137
   Exercises could help avoid a repeat of another Spanish influenza 137
      Exercise #1: Don't ease up on social separating too early 138
      Exercise #2: Young, healthy adults, can be victims of their solid immune systems 140

Exercise #3: Don't toss doubtful drugs at the virus 142

Exercise # 4: Social separating works 143

Exercise # 6: Inoculation works 145

Exercise # 7: Don't blame the sick 147

Exercise # 8: This can end 148

CONCLUSION 149

INTRODUCTION

———— ♦ ◇ ♦ ————

Death was quick, savage, and terrifying. The infection turned victim's bluish-black and suffocated them with their body fluids. The victims would be fine one moment, and crippled and frantic the next, with fevers rising to 104 to 106 degrees. The poor suffered the worst, with the biggest death toll occurring in the slums and tenement districts of huge urban areas; yet it also infected many others.

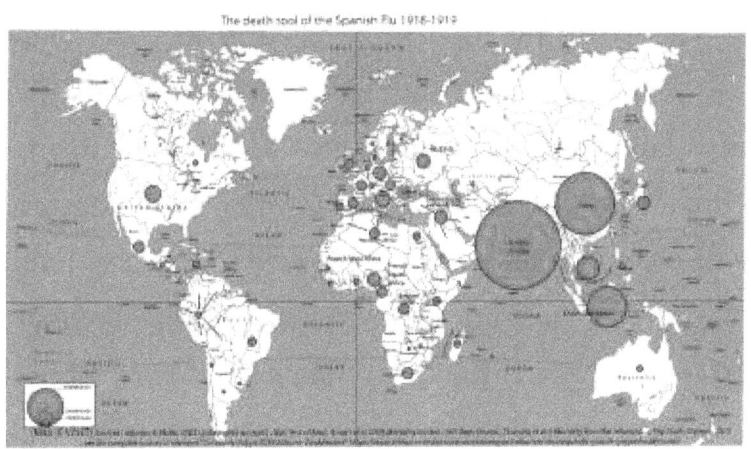

1 - Map F. Vinet[1]

---

[1] Font, N. P. A. S. Johnson, J. Müller, *Updating the accounts: global mortality of the 1918-1920 "Spanish" influenza pandemic*, in Bulletin of the History of Medicine, 2002, 76

The devastation was far more terrible in certain places than others, and history shows hunkering down had an impact. We can relax because of a few favorable circumstances today that show our shielding set up will be considerably more successful than in 1918, when serious minds didn't know humanity would even survive.

At the point when the flu hit in 1918, a few papers detailed that flu represented no risk since it was as old as history; the sort of thing that was generally joined by foul air, fog, and plagues of insects. Advice to residents for preventing illness included keeping their feet dry, remaining warm, eating more onions, and keeping their bowels and windows open. Phonographs were advertised as machines ensured to drive away influenza, because by taking a break tuning in to records, you'd never realize you needed to remain at home around evening time. Even more curious was a portion of the remedies utilized: garlic and camphor balls wrapped by cheesecloth and tied around the necklines; sugar dices saturated lamp oil; formaldehyde tablets, morphine, laudanum, and chloride of lime. Bourbon and Mrs. Winslow's Soothing Syrup, which contained morphine, liquor, alkali were even given to infants and youngsters. The American Medical

Association considered the syrup a "baby killer" in 1911. However, it wasn't removed from the market until the 1930s.

World War I was all the while continuous and wartime restrictions on communication had savage impacts. There were restrictions on writing or publishing anything negative about the country, and banners requested to open "report the man who spreads critical stories." In Philadelphia, specialists convinced reporters to expound on the risk posed to the general population by the Liberty Loan march on September 28, which would gather a large number of individuals who might spread seasonal influenza. Editors would not run the stories or any letters from the specialists. More than 20,000 Philadelphians later passed on of this season's flu virus. When three rushes of Spanish influenza cleared over the globe in 1918 and 1919, in any event, 50 million individuals were dead, including 675,000 Americans. (By examination, influenza pandemics in 1957, 1968 and 2009 claimed an estimated total of 225,000 Americans and 3 million individuals around the world).

CHAPTER 1 - VIRUS' ANALYSIS

---·◇·---

In 1918, a strain of flu known as Spanish influenza caused a worldwide pandemic, spreading quickly and killing indiscriminately. Youthful, old, debilitated, and otherwise healthy people all got infected, and at any rate, 10% of patients died.

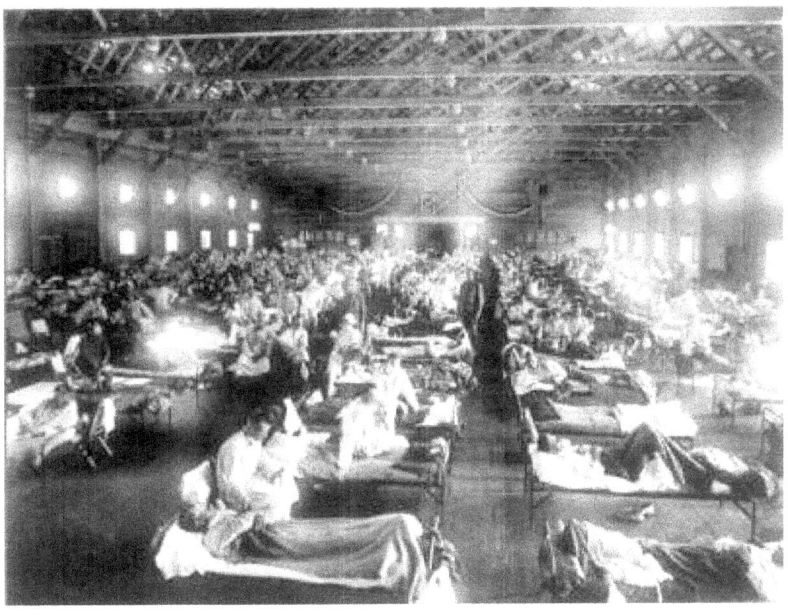

2 - *Emergency military hospital*[2]

---

[2] Camp Funston, Kansas, United States. (Image: courtesy of the National Museum of Health and Medicine, Armed Forces Institute of Pathology, Washington, D.C., United States.)
https://journals.plos.org/plosbiology/article?id=10.1371/journal.pbio.0040050#pbio-0040050-g003

Estimates vary on the specific number of deaths brought about by the disease. However, it is thought to have infected 33% of the total population and killed in any event 50 million individuals, making it the deadliest pandemic in current history. Although at the time it picked up the nickname "Spanish flu," it's unlikely that the virus started in Spain.

What caused Spanish influenza?

The outbreak started in 1918, during the last period of a very long time of World War I, and historians presently accept that the conflict may have been somewhat responsible for spreading the virus. On the Western Front, officers living in cramped, dirty, and damp conditions turned out to be sick. This was a direct result of debilitated safe frameworks from malnourishment. Their diseases, which were known as "la grippe," were infectious, and spread among the positions. Around three days of getting sick, numerous warriors would begin to feel good, yet not all would make it.

Throughout the mid-year of 1918, as troops started to return home on leave, they carried with them the hidden infection that had made them sick. The virus spread across urban areas, towns, and villages in the soldiers' home countries. A large number of those infected, two troopers and civilians, didn't recover quickly. The infection was hardest on youthful adults between the ages of 20 and 30 who had recently been healthy.

In 2014, another hypothesis about the birthplaces of the virus recommended that it previously developed in China, National Geographic reported. Previously undiscovered records connected this season's cold virus to the transportation of Chinese workers, the Chinese Labor Corps, across Canada in 1917 and 1918. The workers were, for the most part, farmworkers from the remote parts of China, as indicated by Mark Humphries' book, "The Last Plague" (University of Toronto Press, 2013). They went through six days in fixed train containers as they were transported across the country over before proceeding to France. There, they were required to burrow channels, empty trains, lay tracks, manufacture streets, and fix harmed tanks. Taking all things together, more than 90,000 doctors were prepared toward the Western Front.

Humphries clarifies that out of 25,000 Chinese workers in 1918, nearly 3,000 finished their Canadian journey in medical quarantine. At that point, and in light of racial stereotypes, their disease was blamed on "Chinese laziness," and Canadian specialists didn't pay attention to the workers' symptoms. When the workers showed up in northern France in mid-1918, many were sick, and hundreds were soon dying.

FOR WHAT REASON WAS IT CALLED THE SPANISH FLU?

Spain was perhaps the earliest country where the plague was recognized. However, history specialists accept this was likely a consequence of wartime censorship. Spain was an unbiased country during the war and didn't uphold severe control of its press, which could consequently freely publish early accounts of the sickness. Subsequently, individuals falsely accepted the disease was explicit to Spain, and the name "Spanish flu" stuck.

Indeed, even in late spring 1918, a Spanish news service reached out to Reuters' London office advising the news organization that "an odd type of sickness of epidemic character has shown up in Madrid. The plague is of a mellow sort, no passing having been accounted for," Inside about fourteen days of the report, more than 100,000 individuals had gotten infected with the flu.

The sickness struck the lord of Spain, Alfonso XIII, alongside leading politicians. Anywhere in the variety of 30% and 40% of individuals who worked or lived in restricted areas, for example, schools, military quarters, and government buildings, became infected. Administration on the Madrid cable car framework must be decreased, and the telegraph service was disturbed in the two cases because there were not enough healthy employees available to work. Clinical supplies and services couldn't stay aware of the interest.

The expression "Spanish flu" quickly grabbed hold in Britain. As indicated by Niall Johnson's book "England and the 1918-19 Influenza Pandemic" (Routledge, 2006), the British press accused this season's flu virus plague in Spain for the Spanish weather: "... the dry, breezy Spanish spring is an upsetting and unhealthy season," read one article in The Times. It was proposed that microbe-laden dust was being spread by the high breezes in Spain, implying that Britain's wet climate may stop the flu from spreading there.

WHAT WERE THE SYMPTOMS OF THE FLU?

Initial symptoms of the sickness incorporated an irritated head and tiredness, trailed by a dry, hacking cough; lost craving; stomach issues; and then, on a subsequent day, extreme perspiring. Next, the disease could influence the respiratory organs, and pneumonia could develop. Humphries clarifies that pneumonia, or other respiratory difficulties achieved by this flu, were regularly the main causes of death. This clarifies why it is hard to decide precise numbers killed by the flu, as the recorded reason for death was often something other than the flu.

By mid-year of 1918, the infection was rapidly spreading to different nations in the terrain of Europe. Vienna, Budapest and Hungary were enduring, and parts of Germany and France were also influenced. Numerous kids in Berlin schools were accounted for as sick and missing from school, and absences in armament factories reduced production.

By June 25, 1918, this flu epidemic in Spain had arrived at the British. In July, the epidemic was striking the London material exchange hard, with one manufacturing plant having 80 out of 400 doctors return home wiped out in one night alone. In London, it covers government workers missing because seasonal influenza goes from 25% to half of the workforce.

The epidemic had quickly gotten to a pandemic, advancing far and wide. Around the same time, cases were accounted for among the Swedish armed force, at that point in the country's civilian population, and among South Africa's working population. By September, this flu had arrived at the U.S. through Boston harbor.

DEVELOPMENT

At the hour of the 1918 pandemic, clinical specialists didn't have any idea about its causes, and toward the start, there were no effective treatments. Before the finish of the pandemic, treatment by transfusion of blood from a survivor was known to be compelling. However, transfusion techniques were simple, performed directly from benefactor to patient, and blood typing and matching were in its beginning.

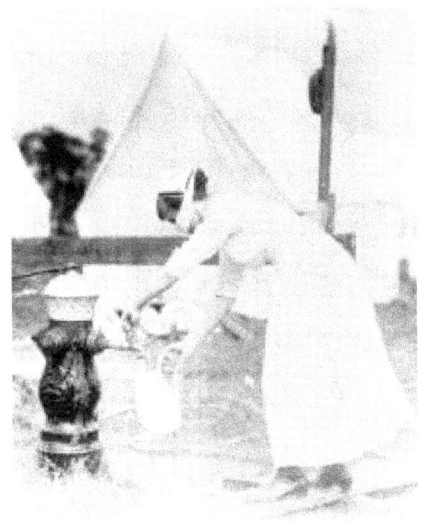

3 - Nurse wearing a mask as protection against influenza. September 13, 1918[3]

Researchers felt that flu was brought about by a bacterium they called Baccilus influenzae (presently

---

[3]Font: http://www.archives.gov/dc-metro/college-park/photographs-dc.htm

known as Hemophilus influenzae.) They could isolate and see numerous sorts of bacteria under a microscope. They additionally realized that there were illness specialists littler than microbes that they could sieve through a mixture. Not having the option to see these exceptionally little specialists, there was a discussion about whether they were chemicals or extremely small organisms. However, vaccines against these extremely small agents, which they called viruses, had just been created returning to the smallpox vaccine in the late 18th century.

In the decades following the pandemic, researchers remembered the risk of flu and attempted to build up a superior comprehension of the sickness. In 1931, Richard Shope considered pigs conveying pig influenza, and applied techniques utilized before decades to identify the reasons for yellow fever and other diseases. He found that the presence of H. flu made swine flu worse, yet didn't cause it. In 1936, Shope indicated that individuals living and dealing with the pig farms had antibodies to pig influenza, demonstrating that the human and swine disease were firmly related. Contemporary scientists created procedures to view such little particles utilizing electron microscopes, and chemically distinguished them as being made up basically of protein and ribonucleic acids.

In 1931, an enormous development was made at Vanderbilt University. Analysts there discovered approaches to develop the flu virus in rich chicken eggs. This meant they no longer needed to get them from sick people or animals. Growing viruses and looking at immunological reactions of lab animals, scientists identified two types of flu infections, called them A and B. The 1918 pandemic infection was a Type A infection. Today we realize that Type A infections infect both people and some different animals and are more dangerous. Type B infections are in humans only.

With the capacity to develop amounts of the viruses, and to identify their qualities, analysts in the late 1930s started working on a vaccine. In 1937, with pressure to get ready for another war developing, British analysts tried a vaccine on officers, and in 1938 the US Army started a trial of vaccines with an exploration group that included Jonas Salk. The first mass utilization of flu vaccines for officers in the United States came in 1944, and for regular people, in 1945. During the exploration of this immunization, it was found that invulnerability against one kind of infection doesn't give immunity against the other. So the vaccine contained a mixture of the two kinds and a point of reference despite everything followed today.

The exploration of the virus, and inoculation to prevent the flu, prompted various disclosures. It made tools for the improvement of different vaccines. Today we, despite everything, utilize ripe eggs to develop infections. It also led to our thoughts on the idea of qualities and the chemicals that encode them. Oswald Avery, an analyst at the Rockefeller Institute, led the group that found in 1944 that deoxyribonucleic acid (DNA) held the genetic code. Their research utilized tools created in recognizing the parts and kinds of viruses and used a bacteria that causes pneumonia. Avery's work was based on the significant work of Frederick Griffith's work that Avery at first set out to disprove. Unfortunately, Griffiths, who was a British researcher, died in the Blitz in 1941.

Although there were attempts at vaccination during the pandemic, the useful adaptation of flu vaccines in the United States started during the 1940s. Thomas Francis Jr. and Jonas Salk, better known later for their work on the polio antibody, were instrumental in the improvement of influenza immunizations. The main approved version of the immunization was controlled to soldiers in 1945, during World War II. Regular folks had the option to get vaccinated the next year.

Flu viruses can transform through antigenic drift and shift, which requires continually adapting vaccine varieties. Since adopting new measures in 1973, the World Health Organization (WHO) decides the three, no doubt flu strains or candidate vaccine viruses (CVVs), to remember for that year's influenza shot. There are likewise quadrivalent immunizations available.

Up to this point, practically all flu vaccines have been fabricated utilizing prepared chicken eggs to propagate the virus. This procedure includes becoming every one of the three anticipated CVVs in separate eggs and joining the three into one vaccine. One of the vital points of attention to this technique is that eggs are less expensive and spread flu to high titers. There are disadvantages, however. In some uncommon examples, the egg-based vaccines have caused allergic reactions. If an avian flu strain were to get harmful, it could crush poultry populations and cause a shortage of eggs for utilization or vaccine manufacturing, which happened in 2015 with the highly pathogenic H5N2. There are presently viral vectored vaccines available now that can help the poultry makers if another H5 episode like this happens; these inoculations uses Charles River's Specific Pathogen Free (SPF) cells or eggs.

In any case, egg-based procedures can be tedious and flighty, with a multi-month slack between CVV segregation and completed immunizations, and changes in the measure of immunization gathered from each egg. In this way, flu vaccine producers are looking for options.

Then again, specialists have been chipping away at cell-based vaccines to replace the standard egg strategy. In 2016, the U.S. Food and Drug Administration (FDA) accepted the production of Novartis' antibody Flucelvax utilizing cell-based virus isolation. In this process, cultured animal cells are utilized to incubate the viruses rather than eggs. This procedure not just eliminates the potential issue of an influenza outbreak, but also allows for faster assembling; however, it is not quicker than traditional techniques where flu in eggs incubates in 48-72 hours.

Since the Spanish influenza emergency, there have been three more flu pandemics, most as of late in 2009. Luckily, since the invention of vaccines and different advances in current social insurance, none have been about as savage as the 1918 pandemic. In any case, without a universal flu vaccine and with certain individuals unfit or reluctant to get a yearly shot, it is just a short time before another outbreak occurs. Flu is a dubious infection and has even stood out as truly newsworthy this year, with new strains being found in dogs. In any case, with continually advancing technologies like cell-based vaccines, future doctors are prepared to set up a fight against the flu.

CHAPTER 2 - ORIGINS AND CAUSES

---◆---

THREE WAVES OF SPANISH FLU

First Wave: Springtime in Spain, 1918

Spain stayed neutral during World War I. As the finish of the war drew nearer in 1918, the country faced a problematic public and political circumstance. Alfonso XIII, the King of Spain, controlled a socially divided country with the vast majority of its near 20,000,000 residents ruined, given the lack of trade and supplies that came about since the beginning of World War I. In Spain, the swelling rate was the utmost (20.1%) it had been since the start of the twentieth century. There was an expanding rate of social class clashes, including a few general strikes.

The first public news of the epidemic showed up in Madrid. On 22 May 1918, the flu scourge was a title text in Madrid's ABC paper. News expressed that the spread of a strange influenza-like illness, which was extremely gentle, had been continuous since the start of May. Due to Madrid's yearly local holidays (Fiesta de San Isidro), an extraordinary number of individuals assembled in assembly halls and well-known gatherings (Verbenas) during the third seven day stretch of May and, in this manner, were likely presented to a high risk of virus transmission. The reported illness was a sudden one; a few people even have fallen while strolling on the road. The ailment introduced as a 2–3-day fever, gastrointestinal side effects, and general anxiety and was related to an exceptionally low death rate. After seven days (28 May), King Alfonso XIII turned out to be sick, as did the Prime Minister and some cabinet members. Many workers remained at home from work given the disease, and some basic services, including the postal and telegraph services, and a few banks and saving accounts offices had to briefly close operations. The plague was day by day news around then, under the feature "La Epidemia refinance" ("The Prevailing Epidemic"). As a result of the perceived lack of severity of the disease and due to Spanish comical inclination, the flu was referred to prominently in Madrid as the "Soldado de Napoles" ("Naples Soldier"), which was the name of a mainstream melody from an exceptionally fruitful melodic, La canción Del Olvido, which was playing simultaneously at Madrid's Teatro de la Zarzuela. The song was well known to such an extent that it was deemed to be "highly contagious," like flu.

A few observers recommended that the pestilence could have been spread from France due to the overwhelming railroad traffic of unskilled Spanish and Portuguese specialists to and from France, who gave transitory substitution to the lack of youthful French workers engaged in the war. Besides a historical competition among France and Spain, this is the likely reason why, in Spain, the flu was otherwise called the French flu. As a result of their regular travel by railroad, these migrant workers were a feasible hotspot for the introduction and spread of the flu infection in Spain. Beginning in focal and southern France (near the battlefields and Army camps) and following the railway way path from north to east (Portugal), and from north to south (Andalusia), the flu spread all through almost the entirety of Spain's areas. Death rates related to flu in this first time of the pandemic extended from 0.04 to 0.65 deaths per 1000 inhabitants. The general death rate increased only slightly during this first plague period. The unknown and elusive etiology of the pandemic further hampered and discredited the work of public health physicians, who were tested day by day by the press. However, the first period of the epidemic was over rapidly. About 2 months after the fact, everything appeared to have returned to ordinary.

Second Wave: Autumn and winter in Spain, 1918

The second time of the pandemic showed up gradually in numerous parts of Spain in September 1918, arriving at its top in October and waning in December 1918.

It is difficult to confirm whether the A (H1N1) virus was reintroduced to Spain from France or whether the virus was all the while circling inside the country. General health authorities acknowledged the significant job that the railway transportation system may play in the spread of the epidemic. Several infection-control measures in fundamental inland train stations and center points were implemented. Trains stacked with Portuguese specialists were halted in Spain, halfway to Portugal, and travelers were not allowed to leave the train until it left again to Portugal. Spanish military preparing camps went about as an efficient diffusion system; sick military workforce with flu were relieved from obligation and sent home via train to rest and get medical care.

When the influenza virus happened in a Spanish town or town, most likely carried there by migrant workers or by military faculty, there was another factor that encouraged its spread. Toward the end of the mid-year, a large number of Spanish towns celebrated their traditional holidays with famous parties and profoundly went to Catholic Mass festivals. In certain cases, flu was even mistaken for foodborne disease, because about the entirety of the people going to these events turned out to be sick a few days later.

Influenza-related mortality rates were very high, extending from 0.5 to 14.0 deaths per 1000 inhabitants. The mean month to month number of deaths of all causes was determined for the period 1913–1917 and was plotted against the watched number of passings for the period September-December 1918. This count gave the excess number of deaths during the second time of the influenza epidemic.

The typical existence of Spaniards was disturbed. School and college terms were canceled, but other public gatherings, for example, those at church services or theaters and films, proceeded. There were hard challenges when trying to execute public health-control measures. Public health officials in Valladolid, Spain, argued with local authorities about officially declaring that there was a progressing plague since local holidays (and the related business) were at their peak. The contention that at last persuaded the authorities included the compensation framework for human service workers. If a physician died of the contamination while on the job and if there was not yet an epidemic circumstance officially declared, at that point, the widow was not qualified for getting a finance benefit from the government. Doctors put the overwhelming focus on the civic chairman of Valladolid, and the flu pandemic was therefore formally announced in Spain.

The town Zamora had one of the most elevated death rates in Spain, arriving at a pinnacle of 10.1% in October 1918 (by and large flu death rate in Spain around the same time was 3.8%). It ranked second to Burgos (flu-related death rate in October 1918 was 12.1%). As a result of a strong social influence of the Bishop, the Catholic Church experts in Zamora expressed that "the evil upon us may be an outcome of our sins and lack of gratitude, and this way the vengeance of eternal justice felt upon us," and hence, organized a progression of Mass social occasions at Zamora's Cathedral. One of the probable outcomes of the events was the easy spread of the infection. The efforts of civil authorities to forbid Mass get-togethers were questioned by the Bishop, who blamed the administrative and public health establishments of excessive obstruction with the church. Every day Mass proceeded with significantly larger audiences in a difficult situation and distress. A typical supplication around then was an old one named Pro tempore pestilentia (For the Times of Pestilence), which asked God that people be saved from plague and starvation, and communicated the individuals' conviction that it was God's will that they were burdened and that God's kindness would end the tribulation.

Public health actions received by political specialists included cleansing with phenolic oil or creoline (Zotal, a popular disinfectant at that point). The Spanish Royal Academy of Medicine asked the foundation and the viability of these techniques; however, the assessment of local authorities prevailed, and travelers, their things, and railroad and tramway wagons were purified. Theaters, cafeterias, and churches were also disinfected. Indeed, even the mail was cleaned. In some Spanish urban areas, avenues were cleaned with a blend of water and sodium hypochlorite, and spitting was restricted. In Madrid, the Congress and the Senate structures were also disinfected.

Doctors and Public Health Officials recommended a few measures to prevent influenza transmission. These measures included cleaning and sanitizing the mouth and nostrils with hydrogen peroxide or a blend of oil and menthol, staying away from gatherings or social occasions in closed settings, avoiding direct contact with sick individuals, eating a healthy diet, frequently walking in new outdoors, ventilating homes, and periodic resting. These simple measures were frequently difficult to watch, particularly for the lowest-income population.

The Spanish Health System was overpowered and didn't give a productive reaction. Numerous little towns spread around the country needed clinical help; their doctors died, and the replacement was difficult (some volunteer clinical school students were deployed).

The little exhibit of medicines recommended included indicative treatment with salicylates and quinine and codeine for cough. For people who created pneumonia, the remedial options were considerably less and included intramuscular or intravenous treatment with silver or platinum colloid arrangements, digitalis, alcamphoroil, or adrenaline. Draining was regularly utilized. Some trial vaccines were additionally attempted, notably those including mixtures of pneumococci, streptococci, and

Pfeiffer bacillus (Haemophilus influenzae). All efforts end up being almost futile, and Spaniards began pondering again whether clinical specialists and researchers had any thought of what was happening.

In light of the high death rate, burial service homes and houses of churches were besieged. Some Spanish urban areas ran out of coffins. The chairman of Barcelona mentioned the military's assistance for the transportation and burial of the dead because city hall workers on the job were scared. Some exceptional laws were confirmed, including the suspension of the standard 2–3-day memorial service functions that drove towards the Dead Mass (Corpore insepulto), which closes with the internment of the body as per the Catholic rites. Corpses were ordered to be buried as quickly as time allows, without the typical long services. Indeed, even the regular church ringer's cost for the dead from the sixteenth century (Toque de difuntos), described by its speeding up, and was restricted in certain towns to avoid further panic and demoralization of the inhabitants. The Spanish papers of that time typically committed the first page or pages to obituaries; during the peak of the second scourge time frame, upwards of 4 or 5 pages were utilized for obituaries.

Third Wave: Winter and spring in Spain, 1919

The third and last time of the influenza epidemic in Spain happened from January through June 1919. The seriousness and length of this period were milder than those of the previous pandemic time frame. It fundamentally influenced the regions of Spain where the principal scourge happened, and it saved most of the areas that were generally influenced constantly. Death rates went from 0.07 to 1.40 deaths per 1000 occupants. The total number of people who died on of flu in Spain were authoritatively assessed to be 147,114 in 1918, 21,235 in 1919, and 17,825 in 1920.

If the common epidemiological index for deaths because of pneumonia and flu is utilized, in light of official morbidity and mortality figures, almost certainly more than 260,000 Spaniards died; nearly 75% of these people died during the second time of the pestilence, and 45% died in October 1918. The mortality design related to the Spanish flu that was seen somewhere else was also found in Spain; death rates were higher among persons aged less than1 year and among those aged 25–29 years.

In general, the death rate in 1918 was the most noteworthy in Spain in the twentieth century. The population growth (net increase of inhabitants) was negative in Spain just twice during the twentieth century: in 1918 (identified with the flu pandemic; net gain, -83.121 people) and in 1939 (identified with the Spanish Civil War; net gain, -50.266 people). The excess mortality related to the 1918-1920 flu pandemic in Spain was 1.49% (95% CI, 1.47%-1.50%).

A few reports recommended that more than 8 million Spaniards developed flu, yet a few Spanish authors dismissed this figure as overestimated. In 1918, a Medical Journal from British advised about this figure: "The flu that we read much about in the everyday papers appears to have been especially far-reaching in Spain during the long stretch of May; that there were 8 million instances of the ailment in that nation, as the French press claimed at that point, is a statement requiring maybe a grain of salt for deglutition; however, it positively highlighted a substantial rate". Considering the broadcast rate in the 1918-1919 Spanish influenza pandemic, it isn't surprising that a high number of people acquired the illness; however, most experienced a gentle and more common clinical presentation. The lack of highly solid morbidity statistics blocks any additionally refined investigation of this information.

A couple of months after its beginning, the presence of the plague was recognized outside Spain: "Flu exists obviously in each country in Europe, and in North, West, and South Africa; in India, as well as in the North American Continent. The commonness pestilence this year came about first in Spain in May. The Canadian Medical Association Journal stated that,, "Under the name of Spanish flu, a pandemic is sweeping over the North American Continent. It is said to have shown up first in Spain, hence called Spanish flu".

The 1918–1919flu pandemic was the worst pandemic that has happened in Spain. It placed remarkable weight on the public health and medical systems and clinical experts. The pandemic was most likely responsible for over 260,000 deaths (1% of the Spanish population), with excess mortality of near 1.5%.

The flu pandemic was referred to worldwide as the Spanish flu. Since the pandemic, Spain has been added to a verifiable short rundown of nations with illness-related names. Albeit a few countries are presently claiming Spanish flu as their own and virologists and disease transmission experts agree that the infection most likely didn't start in Spain, but the 1918 flu pandemic will consistently be known as the Spanish influenza pandemic. Spain and the remainder of the world should always remember the warning that was received.

This flu that transformed the world

Pathologist Jeffery Taubenberger of the US National Institute of Allergy and Infectious Diseases – the man who is 2005, with his associate Ann Reid, published the genetic sequence of the virus liable for the pandemic, said at an ongoing conference that there were as yet numerous unanswered outstanding questions.

Analysts everywhere throughout the world are working to answer them. Yet, what they have just revealed may surprise you.

The fittest were among the most vulnerable

Austrian craftsman Egon Schiele died of flu in October 1918, only a couple of days after his significant other Edith, who was pregnant with their first child, died. Then, desperately sick and grieving, he took a shot at a painting that depicted a family of his own that could never exist.

Schiele was 28 years of age, solidly inside an age group that demonstrated intense helplessness against the 1918 influenza. It is one motivation behind why his unfinished painting, The Family, is frequently depicted as a poignant testimony to the disease's cruelty.

Since it was so dangerous to 20-to-40-year-olds, the disease robbed families of their providers and communities of their columns, leaving huge quantities of old individuals and orphans without any means of help. Men were generally at high risk of dying, compared to the women, except for the ladies that were pregnant, in which circumstance, they died or suffered miscarriages in droves.

Researchers don't know precisely why those in the prime of life were so vulnerable. However, a possible explanation is the fact that the older people, rather than being at a high-risk of dying of influenza, were in reality, less likely to die in the 1918 pandemic because they had been in influenza seasons all through the earlier decade.

One hypothesis that possibly clarifies both observations is "unique antigenic sin," – the possibility that a person's immune system develops its best reaction to the main strain of influenza it experiences. Influenza is a highly labile infection, implying that it changes its structure constantly but remembering that of the two primary antigens for its surface, known by the shorthand H and N, that draw in with the host's immune system.

As per the National Archives, "One-fifth of the world's population was attacked by this destructive virus. Within months, it had killed a bigger number of individuals than some other diseases in written history. This flu afflicted more than 25 percent of the U.S. population. In one year, the normal life expectancy in the United States dropped by 12 years."

For social and economic specialists, the 1918 influenza pandemic and the end of World War 1 marked the start of a complicated set of social, political, and economic events that keep on affecting up till today.

Locally, 1918 marked the end of the "Brilliant Age" of horticulture. Before 1918, the ranch was the social, economic, and political focus in Carroll County.

After World War I, that middle moved to the numerous central avenues of Carroll County's various humble communities. At about a similar time, Westminster was expecting the job of the focal point of an undeniably bureaucratized district government. It was turning into an efficient social, financial, and trade focus.

For numerous historians, the period is mentioned as the "Lost Generation." The term was first begat by Gertrude Stein, who got the thought from her auto specialist. From 1914 through 1918, around 100 million of the people conceived somewhere in the range of 1883 and 1900 passed on from World War I or the flu.

One of the quick consequences of the "Lost Generation" on society was the job of ladies in the public eye was always changed as they left the farms and entered the commercial and mechanical workforce in unparalleled numbers.

As an outcome of the loss or absence of such huge numbers of guys, ladies started to expect leadership roles. They became an economic force that requested investment in settling on community decisions. This dynamic accelerated ladies being given the option to cast a ballot by the nineteenth Amendment in 1920.

The expression "the lost age" has been applied to different groups of individuals who were alive in the mid-twentieth century, including the gifted American artists who came of age during the First World War and the British armed forces officials whose lives were stopped by that war.

In any case, it could reasonably be argued, as I do in my book Pale Rider, that the credit should go to a great many individuals in the principal of lifespan who passed away of the 1918 flu, or to the youngsters who were stranded by it, or to those, not yet conceived, who endured its slings and bolts in their moms' bellies.

The idea of the 1918 pandemic, and of logical information at that point, implies that we don't know precisely what number of people were in those three groups; however, we can be sure that they includeeveryone dwarfed both the Jazz-Age artists and the 35,000-odd British officials who died in combat (South Africa had an expected 500,000 "flu orphans" alone).

The individuals who survived this flu virus in utero in conception lived with the scars until they died. Research suggests that they were less inclined to graduate or earn a reasonable wage, and are bound to go to jail, than peers who hadn't been infected.

What number of people died from Spanish flu?

Exactly 100 years prior, 33% of the world's population found itself infected in a fatal viral pandemic. It was Spanish influenza. Its loss of life is unknown; however, considered to be more than 50 million for the most part.

Some researchers have estimated a death rate as high as 10 to 20%.

During World War I in Europe, influenza struck soldiers and regular citizens in the spring of 1918, and it erupted later in the U.S., where 675,000 individuals passed away.

In the fall of that year, an additional rush of the infection overwhelmed the globe, Bristow said. The youthful and the old were hard hit, yet middle-aged, and in any case, sound people also suffered; those aged 20-40 represented about the portion of the deaths in the pandemic.

"What's noteworthy is this was infectious enough that it seems to have arrived in places for which there's no apparent contact," Bristow stated, referring to an Inuit town in Alaska, where 72 out of 80 inhabitants pass away from the 1918 flu within the span of five days.

Around 50 to 100 million individuals were killed around the world, as indicated by Amesh Adalja, an infectious disease doctor and senior investigator at the Johns

Hopkins Center for Health Security. He puts the passing rate from the 1918 pestilence at around 1 to 2% globally.

Different academics have assessed the death rate from the pandemic to run from 10 to 20%.

All the numbers are best estimates. "In 1918, passing testament recording, and the study of disease transmission was truly in its earliest stages," said Adalja. "We didn't have the entirety of that information. What's more, numerous parts of the world were not associated with different parts of the world. So you couldn't get information from a portion of the poor asset zones that existed around then."

Bristow, Adalja, and different academics generally agree that this season's cold virus pandemic sickened around 500 million individuals.

As much as the medication is battling with the present illness, doctors had even less to challenge with a century back.

"The 1918 pandemic was the most serious pandemic that we have on record," said Adalja. "We had no ICUs around then. We had no vaccines, had no inoculations for flu. We had no clue that this season's cold virus was even a virus around then."

One thing is for sure, and the 1918 pandemic proved that social separating is powerful, as per Bristow.

"In 1918, we applied social separating, however, didn't have a clue about whether it worked or not; presently we know," she said. "It's badly arranged, yet it is the least demanding thing; it's a way that each person can be included and can partake in fighting this virus, and the results will be certain."

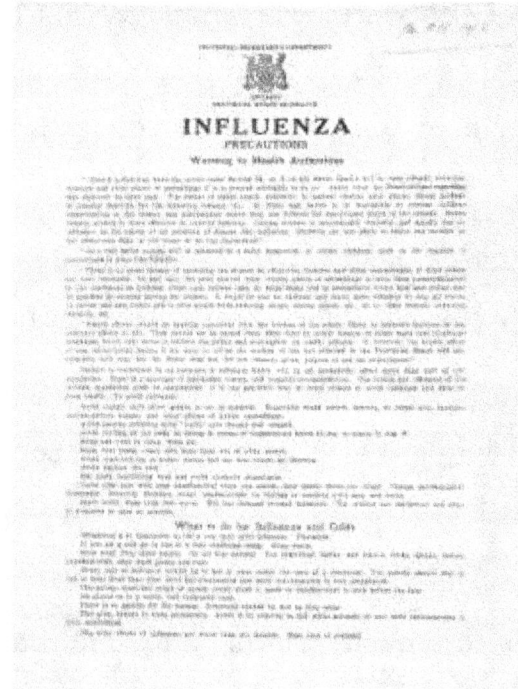

4 - Influenza Poster[4]

---

[4] Font: *Date: October 12, 1918.Creator: Secretary of the Board of Health and Chief Medical Officer of Health subject files..Reference Code: RG 62-4-9-450a.1.Archives of Ontario, I0055101*

CHAPTER 3 - CONSEQUENCES OF VIRUS

—— • ◇ • ——

SPANISH INFLUENZA ORPHANS

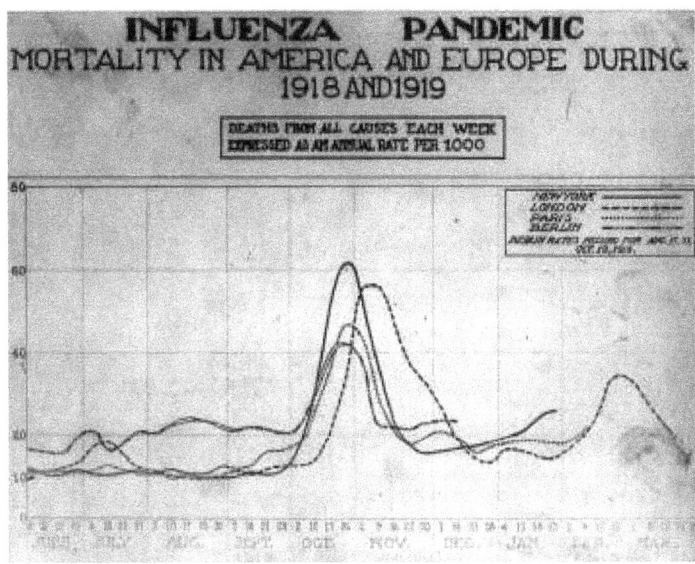

5 - Chart of Mortality[5]

When it decreased in 1920, Spanish influenza had killed 675,000 Americans and left a huge number of children orphaned. Not exclusively accomplished, a greater number of Americans died of Spanish influenza as compared to World War I; more died than in all the wars

---

[5] Chart showing mortality from the 1918 influenza pandemic in the US and Europe
Font: *https://journals.plos.org/plosbiology/article?id=10.1371/journal.pbio.00 40050#pbio-0040050-g003*

of the twentieth century combined. Universally, the pandemic infected 33% of the planet's population and killed an expected 50 million individuals.

However, for all the lives lost and changed forever, Spanish influenza quickly faded from public consciousness. "It fell into this dark hole of history," Davis says. "Affected families never appeared to speak much about it, maybe because it was horrible to such an extent that nobody needed to reconsider it. That is the way the country also dealt with it."

This season's flu virus appeared to hit with a component of randomness, and cruelly so. Since grown-ups in the prime of life died in droves, unlucky communities collapsed. Kids were orphaned, older guardians left to fight for themselves. Individuals were at a loss to clarify this clear lottery, and it left them deeply disturbed. Attempting to portray the feeling it propelled in him, a French specialist in the city of Lyons wrote that it was very dissimilar to the "gut pangs" he had experienced while serving at the front. This was "more diffuse anxiety, the vibe of some indefinable horror which had taken hold of the inhabitants of that town."

It was just later when disease transmission experts focused on the numbers that examples started to rise, and the main components of clarification were advanced. A portion of the variability could be clarified by disparities of wealth and caste, and to the degree that it reflected these factors, as well as skin color. Bad diet, crowded living, and restricted access to human services debilitated the constitution, rendering poor people, settlers, and ethnic minorities more susceptible to disease. As a French student of history, Patrick Zylberman put it: "The infection may well have carried on 'democratically,' yet the general public it attacked was not egalitarian."

Some other underlying diseases made a person more susceptible to Spanish influenza, while earlier presentation to this season's flu virus itself regulated the severity of a case. Remote people group without a lot of verifiable experience of the disease suffered badly, as did urban communities that were bypassed by the first wave of the pandemic since they were not immunologically 'prepared' for the second. For instance, Rio de Janeiro, the capital of Brazil at that point, got just one influx of influenza, in October 1918, and experienced a death rate a few times higher than that recorded in American urban areas toward the north that had gotten both the spring and autumn waves. And Bristol Bay in Alaska was saved until mid-1919, but when the infection at long last increased, it decreased the bay's Eskimo population by 40%.

Public health campaigns didn't have any kind of effect, regardless of the fact that surgeons didn't understand the reason for the disease. Since days of yore, at whatever point disease is a danger, people have polished 'social distancing,' understanding naturally that avoiding infected people builds the opportunity of remaining sound. In 1918, social separating appeared as isolate areas, isolation wards, and prohibitions on mass get-togethers; where they were appropriately upheld, these measures eased back the spread. Australia kept out the harvest time wave altogether by implementing an effective quarantine at its ports.

Similarly dependable, yet in emotional and mental terms, was the grief brought about by the sudden mass death which originated from the pandemic. Families broken by the death of a young parent or companion and orphans, added to the injury spilling out of these deaths, much of the time for the remainder of their lives. In 1998 a ninety-year-old South African influenza vagrant revealed to me that his mom had passed away in the 1918 pandemic when he was ten, "and I have missed her from that point onward. "At the same time a subsequent nonagenarian reviewed powerfully that when his mom had died on of "Spanish" influenza in Illinois in 1918, the sparkle left everything. I understood, just because and forever, that we were not safe. We were not beyond harm. My dad did what he could. He kept us all together, but from that time on, there was a pity which had not existed previously, a where it counts misery that never went away.

In any case, in 1919, most flu widows who had lost their provider husbands had a brief period to harp on their loss, being forced to find immediate approaches to help their youngsters. Going to their families for help, moving into less expensive convenience, or entering the job market more likely than not, had not been an ordinary experience globally for ladies in this circumstance. "My dear spouse kicked the bucket of influenza, leaving me with five youngsters in poverty and debt," conceded one such influenza widow in rustic South Africa. "Petition God for me for acceptance and strength. I intend to go to the diamond diggings to check whether I can get by. Approach the Lord for relief and help. "Many a small scale history will be required before historians can precisely guide such patterns and their variations around the world.

"It was an overall pandemic that took a large number of lives," Troll said. "It reached Alaska, for the most part on the coastal communities. And, had a particularly devastating effect in 1918, in the Nome/Northwest Arctic zone."

But it didn't reach Bristol Bay until 1919, likely because the cannery ships had just left, Troll said. Also, it influenced everyone.

"Local people group, especially in the Northwest and in Bristol Bay, were especially devastated, and a huge crop of orphans were made because of this influenza in both the northwest and in Bristol Bay."

Ringsmuth initiates the NN Cannery history project. The project seeks to preserve the history and experiences of the cannery individuals, from the universal teams to the off-season caretakers.

"This cannery specifically when seasonal influenza pandemic hit Bristol Bay in the spring of 1919, the administrator and the cannery doctor and nurse dealt with the individuals who were caught with Spanish influenza," she said.

Travel in Alaska 100 years prior was, for the most part, by dog sled, and getting health officials into afflicted areas was troublesome, Troll said.

"There was a government doctor in the Dillingham territory, yet this was a wide area, and NN is on the opposite side of the bay," he said. To the credit of the Alaska Packers Association and the whole canning industry in that year, they are the ones that responded and tried to help the individuals who were afflicted, often at risk to themselves."

The pandemic is especially deadly to the adults, which left several kids orphaned by the disease. In the long run, the orphanage was set up close to Dillingham.

"Individuals must have quite recently been overpowered with what was going on," Ringsmuth said. "Most definitely, their large thing was not to allow it to spread."

Isolates were set up to help prevent the spread of the sickness.

"So when they went into the towns, their first intuition was to deal with the individuals who were as yet alive," she said. "At that point, the subsequent stage was to ensure that the bodies were appropriately buried with the goal that the disease wouldn't spread.

Financial effects of the measures taken during the Spanish Flu?

Although there are essential differences between both the economic structures and the actual diseases, it is additionally conceivable to discover similarities; for example, in the policy measures following the two pandemics. Public authorities restricted the free development of individuals a hundred years prior, too, by banning large events and shutting down shops to forestall the spread of the infection. We may, in this manner, take in certain exercises from the emergency brought about by the Spanish Flu on the most proficient method to interpret the consequences of restrictions.

Correia, Luck, and Verner (Opens in another tab) considered the financial impacts of the Spanish Flu and the related non-pharmaceutical interventions in US urban communities. They found that the cities with the highest pandemic mortality experienced the highest reduction in work in the manufacturing industry. The researchers additionally found that if the limitations had been forced sooner and had stayed in power longer, the work rate was higher in the assembling business after the pandemic. The death rate was also lower in these cities.

The outcomes could be interpreted in such a way that, in the short term, governments need to pick between general health and economy. Yet, in the long term, the objectives are no longer contradictory.

The limitations forced during the Spanish Flu accelerated the shock brought about by the pandemic on the economy, yet relieved it later on. A significant exercise to be scholarly may accordingly be that limitations ought not to be viewed as just a method of protecting public health. Still, they ought to also be viewed as tools of fiscal policy.

However, when interpreting the outcomes, it is imperative to remember that the past encounters can't be applied directly to the current circumstance. Also, the death rate; another essential difference between the two pandemics, is the way that the victims of the Spanish Flu were youthful and working-age people. However, the victims of the present seething pandemic are mainly older individuals outside the work power.

As a result of these kinds of differences and different components of vulnerabilities identified with the study, it is of paramount importance to gather quickly as much data as could reasonably be expected on the continuous pandemic. A wide information base empowers financial strategy to be based on a more solid foundation to overcome the crisis.

It is hard to isolate the impacts of the Spanish Flu of 1918-19 from a world previously breaking apart following four years of World War 1.

Thought to have infected 33% of the world's 1.5 billion individuals, the Spanish Flu killed up to 50 million around the world. While the US got off to some degree with a death rate of "just" 0.64%, it despite everything lost around 600,000 individuals, while the UK lost a neighborhood million, and France and Japan 400,000 each. Iran, by and by bearing the brunt of the epidemic, may have lost 2 million individuals, almost 20% of its people.

While policymakers and savants banter the money-saving advantage examination of non-pharmaceutical interventions (NPI, for example, social separating and the close of schools, temples, and organizations), it merits investigating the information from the last worldwide pandemic to decide how lasting its financial impacts.

Since more investigation has been done in the US, our center will place it there. Likewise, the administration and media outlets were hit the hardest, while those gaining practical experience in healthcare products did well.

In the prior days of broadband internet, the other enormous winners were sleeping pad and spring providers, who offered that specialists' best guidance in those days was basically to "remain in bed." Contrast this with today, where the physicians' instructions are to observe bunches of TV, and it isn't hard to imagine which parts will at least momentarily shine.

The death rates and hence the immediate monetary effect were far higher in certain American people group: to be specific thick polluted urban conditions and places where workers were in close contact with each other.

Mining towns were especially hard hit, with the town of Coalfield, Tennessee detailing at the height of the emergency in the fall of 2018 that just 2% of the town was "well." Population densities were also to blame. Although the US was just 51% urban in 1918, compared with 82% today, it had a normal 4.53 individuals for every family unit, the normal size of which was 100sqm (compared with 220sqm today). Also, open wide mobility within the city was less intense.

What, at that point, were its effects?

Much the same as the Black Plague and so many epidemics before and ever since, the Spanish Flu drove up wages, especially in manufacturing. The paper by the St Louis Fed likewise found a huge connection between statewide death rates and ensuing per-capita salary growth by 1930.

A later paper by the Federal Reserve Bank of New York demonstrated that urban communities that intervened before and all the more aggressively observed a greater recovery once the pandemic passed, including "relative increases in assembling business, fabricating yield, and bank resources." As far as assembling goes at that point, lost ground was made up. Over the world, in any case, a paper prior this year from Barro et al. found that higher mortality during the Spanish Flu brought down genuine GDP by 6-8% in affected countries.

Although economies suffered the Spanish Flu greatly, the financial pain despite everything failed to measure up with the impacts, what's more, with the aftermath of World War I.

However, ostensibly the greatest long haul impact may have been with those considered during the epidemic. An ongoing report from Columbia and the National Bureau of

Economic Research has demonstrated that "flu-born cohort" achieved lower instructive fulfillment, had expanded rates of physical inability, lower lifetime wages, and a lower in general financial status than those conceived previously or after the flu.

As the world ponders the wellbeing and monetary outcomes, the 1918 Spanish influenza is getting renewed attention. And, with reason: Spanish influenza affected around 500 million individuals worldwide and killed around 50 million lives, including around 675,000 Americans, or about 0.67% of the country's population. Quite a bit of existing economic work on the flu pandemic has focused on understanding its effect on health and human capital. Considering the sizable immediate contraction in economic activities made by the pandemic outbreak, there is renewed interest in assessing the economics of the 1918 flu pandemic. There was impact of flu-related deaths in 43 countries in 1918-1920 and consequently, higher flu death rates led to declines in GDP and utilization by about 6%. Other work has focused exclusively on the United States. Exploiting spatial variation in death rates, regions in the US that were hit by the pandemic experienced a sharp decrease in financial movement, and the impacts persisted until at any rate, 1923.

While interesting comparisons across countries or urban communities in the US form one remarkable component of the 1918 pandemic, the Spanish flu left practically no discernible mark on the aggregate US economy. On the other hand, the flu outbreak in the spring of 1918 happened directly after a downturn: the Dow Jones Industrial Average had declined by 21.7% in 1917. However, the stock market recovered substantially during the pandemic, with the Dow file expanding by 10.5% in 1918 and by 30.5% in 1919. Indeed, 1919 stands as the ninth greatest year for the Dow from 1915 to 2019. As per a few evaluations, the real gross national product developed in 1919, but by a modest 1%. In new work, markers of aggregate economic activity suffered modestly, and those that declined all the more fundamentally directly after the flu outbreak, as industrial output, recovered within months. That the effect of the flu pandemic on the total US economy was gentle ought to be surprising. As opposed to a current pandemic, which is disproportionately serious for older adults, the Spanish flu was remarkably lethal for those in their 20s and 30s; as it were, those in prime working age. The economy did, in the long run, go into recession in 1921, but by then, the decrease in output had all to do with a breakdown in item costs when post-war European production finally recovered.

The expectation for the immediate economic fallout of the current pandemic is appalling. Experts today expect a staggering 20-30% decrease in GDP for Q2 2020, just as a 15% jobless rate. Also, the Dow lost over 36% of significant worth from its top in February 2020 to its worst point on 23 March 2020, however it has recovered somewhat since then.

So for what reason is the present emergency having such a huge effect on the economy, while Spanish influenza didn't? One potential clarification lies in the social separating measures that the US and different countries have guided to smooth the bend and hinder the spread of the infection. While numerous employments should now be possible remotely from home, many can't. Social removal also cuts the interest of many goods and services. Therefore, a few divisions in the economy have stopped.

However, even in 1918, local governments executed similar limitations on open social occasions to contain the infection. For example, in 1918, the Commercial and

Financial Chronicle, a main business news outlet around then, announced: "In Boston, the subject of shutting the holy places is being talked about as a means of checking the pandemic. In Pennsylvania, all spots of public amusement, schools, holy places, and the total of what cantinas have been requested shut until further notice." And Dr. Rupert Blue, the then-Surgeon General of the US, expressly considered these closings "the best way to prevent the spread of the infection." As it is today, constraining social cooperation was also the key system to slow down contagion more than a century ago.

Regardless, these social separating measures didn't approach those implemented in the US today. Work in factories, mines, and shipyards proceeded, regardless of probably a portion of this work encouraging the spread of the disease. Why? Since organizations were under pressure by the US government to satisfy interest for items and products that were required for the war effort. This carries us to the principle motivation behind why the US economy didn't enormously contract in 1918 WWI.

At the point when the pandemic unfolded, a significant share of the country's assets at home and abroad were given to the war economy. Real government spending represented about 38% of GDP. Indeed, even human capital was, to a great extent, attached to the war effort. By 1918, the military included right around 3,000,000 million sailors, soldiers, and marines, representing up to 6% of the work power between the ages of 15 and 44. As the Chronicle put it, "Towering over each other type of exchange action is the vast business in a hundred roads of the industry to supply the needs of the United States Government and Allied Powers in these earth momentous days." In the interim, regular citizen business was considered as "strictly auxiliary." The increase in the government's interest in war-related items more than compensated for the contraction in buyer spending and private investment.

It is not essentially the case that the 1918 pandemic had no financial outcomes. The Chronicle also reports that coal yield "was extensively decreased by the quick spread of flu in different segments of the country; notably in Pennsylvania, Alabama, Kentucky, Tennessee, Virginia, West Virginia and Maryland," while material plants "whine that they are having great difficulty in keeping up creation." Those urban communities and states that accomplished higher death rates saw a bigger decrease in manufacturing output by about 18%.

But the never-ending demand for coal, steel, hardware, materials, and different items required for the war effort and the impacts of such a serious pandemic had effect on the aggregate economic activity. The private sector continued pushing in requests to satisfy the war-related interest regardless of the shortage of work, as workers turned out to be sick. For example, the Chronicle reports that "with an end goal to help creation, 70,000 coal miners in focal Pennsylvania bituminous coal fields have cast a ballot to work Sundays to conquer lost creation because of flu plague." The government was purchasing; thus firms kept on producing.

What exercises would we be able to gather from the 1918 pandemic for now? We are not pushing for another war, or that laborers be urged to work in unsafe conditions that may elevate their exposure to the virus. But, it is helpful to recall that a worldwide pandemic doesn't inevitably lead to a grave economic recession or depression. More specifically, an enormous development in government requests can go far in relaxing the monetary effect of a crisis that takes steps to lessen utilization and private investment.

Reviewing the Spanish Flu: 'We ought to gain from our mistakes'

Although it feels like we're experiencing an exceptional emergency right now, Concord, similar to a significant part of the remainder of the world, experienced something fundamentally the same a century before the infection that came to be known as the Spanish Flu.

"You perceive how rapidly the medical clinics in Concord were overpowered. The Elks Club expanding on Main Street was transformed into a crisis clinic and set up with visiting medical caretakers and volunteers," said Byron Champlin. He has focused on how the 1918-1919 worldwide pandemic influenced Concord. City authorities in Concord in late September of 1918 shut down basically wherever individual congregated – theaters, hair parlors, soft-drink shops, cantinas. Holy places ended Sunday services, and they closed the schools down. Fraternal associations, book clubs, most reported that they were suspending social affairs. In the long run, the Board of Health guided just close family to go to burial services."

Sound natural? This does as well: Until it couldn't be ignored, officials underplayed the seriousness, Champlin said.

"There were little things in the paper in those days, frequently placed without attribution. They would make statements like 'This is only the grippe, simply the normal grippe,'" he stated, utilizing an old term for a cold or influenza. "It's striking that the Hopkinton Fair went on as usual in September, with around 3,700 people gathered there."

The disease emerged in the U.S. in the fall of 1918, as the country was fighting hard in World War I. Authorities cinched down on references to the epidemic, fearing it would undermine efforts in the war, which finished in November 1918. Simply after the war finished, did news come increasingly across the board.

For instance, Champlin highlighted banks.

"They were extending hours so individuals could come in and purchase war bonds," he said. "Some portion of the feeling that you would not like to do anything to inhibit on war confidence."

"It wasn't till the illness at the top in Concord that you saw real activity," he included.

Amateur historian

Champlin, of Concord, says he has "consistently been an amateur historian" and, in the wake of resigning from the protection business and philanthropic work, needed to write a history of Concord in World War I. That is the point at which he understood the seriousness of the Spanish Flu.

"There are 43 labels of war passed away on the landmark in Memorial Field. Five passed away from the disease, 3 of them of flu," he said. "Indeed, even the battlefront is connected."

Around the world, it's evaluated that the Spanish Flu, a variation of the H1N1 infection that caused a littler pandemic in 2009, killed somewhere close to 20 million and 100 million individuals – in any event, 1% and maybe as much as 4% of the whole worldwide population at that point. The death estimation in the US was supposed to be 675,000, although that is highly uncertain.

It's not so much clear where the 1918 pandemic began; however, it spread when individuals contacted each other.

A significant purpose of transmission through New Hampshire was Fort Devens's army base in Massachusetts. In this significant wartime activity, a large number of fighters and others traveled every way even as the illness produced brutality, and spread.

The sickness is called Spanish Flu since Spain was the main country in Europe lacking controls on papers during the war. Press opportunity implied that as the sickness was developing, Spain was the main spot that kept announcing about it.

Not much reporting

Writing about the pandemic was practically nonexistent in the United States during the war in light of press restrictions, which clarifies why this national disaster has been somewhat forgotten.

"There are no photographs that I've had the option to discover of anything occurring in Concord during the pandemic," said Champlin. Paper reports of the time are crude until after it became a full-blown epidemic, and histories of the time frequently portray the disease for the most part, as a short-term irritant.

The Granite Monthly, a magazine devoted to "writing, history and state progress" of New Hampshire, has no articles about the ailment in the bound edition of its 1918 publications. "Flu" is referenced just every so often, for example, to clarify why the Congregational Church didn't hold its centennial celebration on schedule or why a Food Administration Booth asking individuals to save food in wartime now and again drew little groups. "The full efficiency of the stand was delayed by the flu scourge," the magazine noted, before talking about the utilization of "light slides" in cinemas to get the food-conservation message.

"You realize how battle veterans don't care to discuss their experiences? I think anyone who endures the flu would not generally like to discuss it. The thinking was, we have to proceed onward," Champlin said.

Champlin wrote a long piece published in the Monitor in September 2018, the centennial anniversary of the disease truly striking home. He arranged all the accounts of history that he could discover.

"It was rehashed ordinarily in the news sections of the Monitor, of relatives passing away within days of each other. There were a few twofold memorial services. It's heartbreaking."

That sort of distress, worsened by ignoring the issue until it was past the point of no return, is the reason Champlin believes it's critical to remember the last time the world reeled due to a virus.

"From my point of view, it's significant for individuals to see how serious this sort of thing can be," he said. "We ought to gain from our mistakes."

The Spanish flu in Kingston

Kingston experienced one of the most noteworthy influenza-related death rates in Canada, with various elements adding to the local pandemic. Kingston was a military center, and many returning soldiers were either positioned at or sifted through the city. Adding a health complication to the previously overpowering assignment of returning troopers home, the flu forced many soldiers to broaden their stay in Kingston before they were allowed to travel again.

Moreover, Kingston boasted two clinics that had the option to help numerous evil patients from different networks: Kingston General Hospital and Hotel Dieu Hospital. During the pandemic, these changeless clinics were supported by temporary emergency clinics all through the city.

A hospital named as Queen's Military had opened in the new expressions building (presently Kingston Hall) and Grant Hall from the get-go in 1917 to help ease crowding at KGH, which around then, had patients remaining in the lobbies. The Queen's clinic held 600 beds between the two buildings. When Spanish influenza hit in the fall of 1918, the Queen's Military Hospital started to fill in as a flu hospital as well.

The most critical factor that added to the high in-emergency clinic demise rate in Kingston was that treatment in the medical clinic was free. In contrast to most emergency clinics in the area, Kingston had a remarkable connection between the Queen's clinical school and KGH. Free patient confirmation empowered hands-on learning for medical students while urging individuals to look for help at hospitals as opposed to remaining at home. —This empowered individuals from encompassing networks to venture out to Kingston for their care.

Following primary influenza outbreak in Kingston on October 7 because of pneumonia, individuals started to develop a more significant appreciation for the especially detrimental results of that year's influenza. With more than 33% of its staff sick, The Daily British Whig was experiencing difficulty finishing its delivery routes because huge numbers of the course runners had gotten this season's cold virus. Two compositors at the paper were also sick, bringing about notices running a few days straight without changeover.

Meanwhile, Bell Telephone's workplaces in Kingston and somewhere else were short-staffed. With one-third of its employees, Bell mentioned that the open make just crisis calls until staff recovered. The Kingston, Portsmouth, and Cataraqui Street Railway had 10 employees, four of them conductors, become sick with flu, requiring significant adjustments to the train schedule.

Every nearby leading group of health could close public places. On October 4, the close by town of Renfrew shut its schools, weapons manufacturing plant, and a few other modern organizations after five revealed deaths from flu. After fourteen days, and with the pandemic worsening, the choice was made in Kingston to close down all schools and open places in the city.

While this choice was challenged, particularly by business owners whose livelihoods were legitimately influenced by the closures, others exploited the circumstance. Treadgold's Sporting Goods encouraged Kingstonians to buy one of their phonographs and remain safe and entertained at home. Also, O'Connor's apparel store guaranteed its customer base that the store was disinfected every day, guaranteeing stress-free looking for deals.

The more than multi-week term following October 16, 1918, remains the main time that Queen's University has been shut for a medical reason. During this time, a considerable lot of the students returned home to think about friends and family and escape the close quarters of Queen's lodging. Nursing and medical students were constrained to remain and help in the overpowered neighborhood and close by medical clinics. About a large portion of the medical students remained in Kingston; the other half were dispatched to surrounding regions, from close by Gananoque and Madoc to as distant as Collingwood and Sherbrooke.

The Queen's Military Hospital had 141 confirmations between October 7 and 21. At the point when it turned out to be certain that influenza cases would dwarf the accessible beds at KGH, Hotel Dieu Hospital, and the Queen's Military Hospital, an extra crisis medical clinic was set up on Princess Street at the Great War Veterans' Association. Opening on October 19, the medical clinic thought about ladies and kids experiencing flu. Individuals from 22 families were conceded with a sum of

57 patients, two of whom were kids who died during their stay.

In a shockingly organized effort, the Provincial Board of Health started the Ontario Emergency Volunteer Health Auxiliary (OEVHA). The OEVHA held lectures in cities all through the province to prepare ladies as volunteer emergency nurses. The individuals who passed the short course were given a uniform with the badge "ONTARIO S.O.S." (Sisters of Service). In Kingston, 156 ladies chipped in for the Sisters of Service more than 18 days, with 1,255 home visits being made to 200 families, seeing an aggregate of 600 patients.

Although the college was closed for 18 days starting on October 16 the Queen's people group remained very dynamic during this period. As detailed in the Queen's Journal on November 5, "Sovereign's students have taken phone messages for the specialists; Queen's students have given a clinical guide where doctors have been too occupied to even think about going; Queen's students nursed the sick, by day and around evening time, in crisis emergency clinics, in military medical clinics, and private homes; Queen's students have run S.O.S. vehicles; they have set up lunches for nurses; they have assumed responsibility for stores and workplaces to discharge others for S.O.S. work; they have assisted with extremely difficult work in the cemeteries; anyplace, what's more, everything along the line Queen's understudies have been pushing out, up over the top, and against this thing that has been eating its path eagerly over our property."

THE SEARCH FOR A VACCINE

At the point when influenza hit eastern North America in the fall of 1918, the possibility of immunization as a treatment was at that point in the brains of numerous scientists. However, there were advantages to having various vaccines produced at the same time, and this made it trying for health practitioners to figure out which, assuming any, to give patients. Most vaccines available professed to be preventative, while a couple of additionally proposed remedial worth. Given the sheer number of choices available to doctors, many chosen to utilize antibodies if all else fails, despite their preemptive worth.

Guilford Reed was a lecturer at Queen's at that point, first in the Department of Biology and afterward in the Department of Pathology and Bacteriology. On October 1,

1918, Dr. Reed started looking into a potential vaccine by taking nasopharyngeal swabs of 70 patients with flu. He broke down the swabs for their bacterial substance and found that 94 percent of the swabs had Bacillus influenzae (present-day Haemophilus influenzae type b); 50 percent Pneumocococci; 56 percent "green-delivering" Streptococci (current Streptococcus pneumoniae); and 31 percent Moraxella catarrhalis. From the microbial classes, ten strains of B. influenzae and Pneumococci, alongside five strains of Streptococci and M. catarrhalis were developed in pure cultures on agar with rabbit's blood.

From these isolates, Dr. Reed built up an antibody and prophylactically inoculated 193 medical students, 142 of whom got three dosages of his invention. The most encouraging outcome he watched was that more than 45 percent of unvaccinated people gotten this season's cold virus, while just 12 percent of vaccinated people became sick.

Despite the guarantee of Dr. Reed's work, his exploration didn't prompt any significant treatment protocol changes. The pandemic, although devastating, was genuinely transient, and it was over before specialists and doctors could respond adequately. Also, it was trying to create an enormous amount of vaccines in such a brief timeframe.

Tragically, Dr. Reed's work was uncertain and unfit to show worthy adequacy to push ahead rapidly.

Although numerous specialists worked tirelessly to build up an effective bacterial vaccine, future research featured how far away they had been. Although the contrasts among microscopic organisms and infections were starting to be understood, the significant qualifications were not yet valued. Microbes are progressively self-ruling single-celled life forms that are altogether bigger than infections, which require a host to infect. It was not until 1933, when all the more impressive microscopes revealed the size difference, that the genuine viral starting points of flu got known.

How the 1918 Flu Pandemic Helped Shape Respiratory Care

One hundred years prior this year, the deadliest pandemic influenza the world has ever observed cleared far and wide, contaminating about 33% of the total population and killing around 20 to 50 million individuals, incorporating around 675,000 in the U.S.

First seen in Europe, America, and regions of Asia, the illness came to be known as the "Spanish Flu," likely because Spain was especially hard to hit and was not dependent upon the World War I news power outages that kept the expression of the disease in different countries from getting out.

Previously healthy young people were disproportionally affected, with authorities assessing 40 percent of U.S. Naval force service members, and 36 percent of those in the Army get the disease.

Research led in 2008 at long last clarified why the 1918 influenza was so deadly: a gathering of three qualities empowered the infection to debilitate the bronchial cylinders and lungs and led to bacterial pneumonia that at last took such a large number of lives.

Wakeup call

AARC Historian Trudy Watson, BS, RRT, FAARC, who just made a new gallery for the AARC's Virtual Museum including the pandemic, says the 1918 outbreak was a reminder for health care professionals.

"A considerable lot of the essential exercises gained from the 1918 flu pandemic are reflected in common practice today: covering coughs, visit hand washing as well as utilizing hand sanitizers, and utilizing suitable personal protective equipment," Watson said.

She notes surveillance projects to screen the number and area of flu cases developed after the 1918 flu episode also, and a portion of the practices that were set up to battle the spread of this season's cold virus in those days are still being used today.

"As in 1918 when schools, church services, and other network exercises were dropped in the expectation of decreasing the spread of flu, we saw similar temporary closures in communities where influenza cases were common during the ongoing 2017-2018 influenza season," says Watson.

Those preventative estimates overflow to human services offices as well.

"Numerous human services offices demoralize and limit guests at the pinnacle of influenza season to limit transmission and firmly urge staff to stay at home if they experience flu side effects," she said.

The new spotlight on antibodies

Maybe the hugest progression to come out of the pandemic, in any case, was another emphasis on the development of vaccines that could keep the sickness from happening. While quite a few years would go before these vaccines and other treatments like antibiotics would be prepared for open use, the ball was gotten underway.

The main influenza immunization went ahead of the market in 1938 and was immediately trailed by different antibodies and anti-microbial: streptomycin for the treatment of tuberculosis in 1944, penicillin in 1945, the pertussis antibody in the late 1940s, and the polio immunization in 1952.

"Most of these operators opened up just as inhalation therapy was rising as a calling," Watson said. "Early inhalation therapy practitioners and doctors cooperated to present new treatment modalities, develop hardware, and implement disease prevention techniques."

RTS are key players

A considerable lot of those treatment modalities were driven by pulmonary pioneer Dr. Alvan Barach, whose enthusiasm for clinical oxygen treatment was started by experiences he had while seeing the treatment of influenza patients during his clinical preparation in 1918-1919.

As he told Dr. Tom Petty, in a 1979 meeting, when it created the impression that patients were 10 or 15 minutes from death, he saw doctors hold a channel about an inch away from their appearances into which oxygen has risen from a low-pressure tank. While the youthful doctor noticed no advantage from this last-ditch effort, it made him consider whether oxygen could be viable with higher concentrations.

Dr. Barach's examination, combined with that of different pioneers in the field, prepared for the key pretended by respiratory therapists in the fight against the yearly episode of flu today. In addition to the fact that therapists are essential to the consideration delivered to individuals who are hospitalized with the condition, they additionally help instruct their patients, the general population, and even their associates about the requirement for the annual flu vaccine.

"At the point when the 1918 flu outbreak began, influenza vaccines just didn't exist," Watson said. "Today, the CDC suggests that everybody more than a half year get an annual flu vaccine. Health care professionals are supported, and as a rule, required to get an annual flu vaccine for employment."

"In those days, it was not exactly as clear how sicknesses like flu were transmitted and what should be possible to decrease transmission," said Parada.

In 1918, in a couple of urban communities where sorted out measures were founded to confine irresistible illness outbreaks, the spread of the Spanish influenza was a lot of lower, Parada said. Measures we take presently incorporate the frequent washing of hands, covering the nose and mouth in the wake of sneezing, avoiding touching the eyes, nose, and mouth, and utilizing disinfectants on as often as possible touched surfaces where germs can wait.

"In many spots that weren't finished, there was almost no push to block transmission, and those individuals followed through on the cost," Parada said.

Essentially, the Spanish influenza pandemic happened before the appearance of antibiotics, which are powerful in treating secondary infections brought about by the flu, Parada said. A large number of the deaths that happened during the 1918 pandemic were the results of secondary bacterial infections called post-flu pneumonia.

"It was the pre-antibiotic age. If you had post-flu pneumonia, the probability of doing ineffectively and dying on was a lot higher," Parada said. "We're in the anti-toxin age now, and we improve employment of treating and preventing post-influenza pneumonia."

Furthermore, in 1918 those tainted with the Spanish flu didn't approach the propelled care and technology standard in serious consideration units over the country, Parada said. Without the guide of ventilators, for example, victims of the 1918 pandemic who advanced to respiratory failure invariably died.

"They didn't have ventilators, so they passed on," Parada said. "Rather than respiratory failure being a death sentence as it was in 1918, we can get you past the halfway point until you react to treatment and the ventilator are removed."

Additionally, in contrast to 1918, there are two doctor prescribed medication that is viable against the H1N1 influenza strain – Tamiflu (an oral prescription) and Relenza (a breathed in drug). The federal and state governments have stockpiled a huge number of portions of the two meds for crisis use.

"The prior treatment is begun, and the more compelling it is," Parada said. "If treatment is begun following 72 hours of symptoms, it has exceptionally restricted impact. It has a greater effect if it's begun following 48 hours and a far superior impact if it's begun within 24 hours of symptoms."

Even better, Tamiflu and Relenza can both be utilized to prevent infections, Parada said. This is called prophylaxis treatment.

"We try to limit the utilization of prophylaxis to unique conditions, particularly in instances of people weakened by cancer, transplant, or HIV. The medicines can stop flu infections from really developing," Parada said. "These treatments are also used to treat medicinal services laborers who inadvertently become infected at work. We can't have every one of our laborers becoming ill, missing work or more awful yet, coming to work sick and tainting our patients."

In any case, the best treatment for this season's cold virus is anticipation, Parada emphasized

"I am a strong supporter of everybody getting the yearly seasonal flu shot, and once the H1N1 vaccine opens up, I suggest that all high-risk patients get that vaccine too," Parada said.

Those patients incorporate pregnant ladies, family unit contacts and parents for youngsters more youthful than a half year, human services and emergency medical services staff, individuals from ages a half year through 24, individuals ages 25 through 64 years who have health conditions related with a higher risk of medical complications from influenza.

CHAPTER 4 - SPANISH FLU TREATMENTS

———— • ◇ • ————

Treating the 1918 Spanish flu was regularly to a greater degree a speculating game than a hard science: individuals took a stab at everything from home remedies to combinations of oils and herbs. Generally, treatment was symptomatic and reactionary. It was popular for individuals to take cinnamon, as oil with milk or as a powder, to help lower the body's temperature. If that failed, Aspirin was usually utilized, which would help with following headaches too. Cyanosis went with certain cases, and this was treated by giving patients breathing devices or infusing oxygen under the skin. A large number of flu cases that resulted in pneumonia were treated with epinephrine.

Strange and ineffective treatments abounded as urgent individuals clung to the idea that something may help. A prime case of this was salt with quinine, a common medication for malaria at that point, which individuals utilized as a flu treatment. Numerous quinine medications contained laxatives, as it was falsely accepted that flushing the framework would help rid the body of disease.

Despite the high number of ineffectual medicines, there was one respectably successful thought: blood transfusions. Although the reason was not completely understood at that point, doctors perceived that expelling the serum from recovering patients and transfusing it into sick patients would help increase survival rates. After the thickening variables, and white and red blood cells, were removed, the rest of the serum comprised of electrolytes, antibodies, antigens, and hormones, which helped sick patients.

Early execution of treatment was basic, as transfusion inside four days of pneumonia difficulties brought about a 19% casualty rate compared to 59% for those standing by longer than four days. The utilization of transfusions took off during the First World War with the guide of three recent discoveries: the existence of differing blood classifications, the utilization of the anticoagulant sodium citrate, and the utilization of refrigeration to store blood. As a final desperate attempt for some patients, transfusions created surprisingly effective results.

Antibody Development over the US

At the Naval Hospital on League Island, Pennsylvania (the Philadelphia Naval Shipyard), doctors portrayed their way to deal with a vaccine: "After the idea of a suffocating individual getting a handle on at a straw, a stock flu vaccine was utilized as a preventive in fifty individual cases and as a corrective specialist in fifty other simple cases." They made the vaccine produced using B. influenzae and strains of pneumococcus, streptococcus, staphylococcus, and Micrococcus catarrhalis (presently Moraxella catarrhalis). Each portion contained somewhere in the range of 100,000,000 and 200,000,000 microorganisms for every cubic centimeter, in a four-dose regimen. The examiners announced that no vaccinated people (who were emergency hospital workers) became sick, but also noticed that strict preventive measures were taken, for example, the utilization of covers, gloves, etc. In a gathering of sick patients treated therapeutically with the antibody, none developed pneumonia, but one developed pleurisy (contamination of the coating of the lungs). They noticed, "The course of the illness [in those treated therapeutically]... was certainly shortened, and adoration appeared to be less extreme. The patients not profited were those admitted from four to seven days after the beginning of their sickness. These were messed up with regards to the number of pneumonia that developed and the severity of the infection of the control cases. The impacts were in every case all the more striking, the moment the vaccines was managed." Finally, they presumed that "The quantity of patients treated with antibodies and the number immunized with it is too little even to consider allowing of certain deductions; yet so far as no untoward outcomes go with their utilization, it would appear to be unquestionably safe and even advisable to suggest their usage."

Another gathering of examiners described the utilization of vaccines at the Naval Training Station in San Francisco. They observed that Spanish flu didn't reach San Francisco until October 1, 1918, and that that staff at the preparation station in this manner had the opportunity to get ready preventive measures. Isolation was simple, because of the area of the base on Alameda Island, which was reachable just by boat from San Francisco and Oakland. Maritime Yard staff were required to utilize a germ-free throat spray daily. Apart from these measures, the authors noticed that "means were taken to deliver a prophylactic vaccine," although there was a "great diversity of feeling concerning the energizing reason" of the pandemic. By and large, pneumococcus and streptococcus were viewed as the reason for the most severe complications. Also, and amid the difference, they chose to acquire a culture of B. influenzae from a lethal case at the Rockefeller Institute to utilize for the vaccine. Taking all things together, the vaccine contained B. influenza, 5 billion microscopic organisms, pneumococcus Types I and II, 3 billion each; pneumococcus Type III, 1 billion; and Streptococcus hemolyticus (S. pyogenes), 100 million.

Guinea pigs were first infused with the antigen to survey harmfulness, and afterward, five lab specialist volunteers were inoculated. Lab tests discovered that their white cell tally also expanded, their sera agglutinated B. influenzae (implying that they had vaccines in their blood that responded to the microscopic organisms). Symptoms from the injection included neighborhood expansion and pain but no abscesses. Offered consent to continue, more vaccine was prepared, and 11,179 military and regular folks were vaccinated, including some at Mare Island (Vallejo, CA) and San Pedro just as San Francisco regular citizens related with the Naval Training station. In most experimental groups, the pace of flu cases was lower than in the uninoculated groups (however no data is given on how the statistics for the uninoculated groups were gathered, nor is their data on how a case was characterized). Also, individuals who were inoculated got the injections around three weeks after flu showed up in California, so it's difficult to tell whether they had just been exposed and infected. The percent of flu cases in control groups ranged from 1.5% to 33.8% (the last being medical nurses in San Francisco clinics), though somewhere in the range of 1.4% and 3.5% (the last being hospital corpsmen on the job in a flu ward) of those in the inoculation group turned out to be sick with flu.

Another utilization of vaccine was archived in Washington State at the Puget Sound Navy Yard. Investigators guarantee that the flu attacked the Navy Yard when a gathering of mariners showed up from Philadelphia (it's unclear precisely when they showed up; however, the paper expresses that "the time of perception was from September 17 to October 18, 1918"). Altogether, 4,212 individuals were vaccinated with a streptococcal vaccine. The investigators revealed that the flu attack rate in the vaccinated varied from 2% to 57% and in the unvaccinated from 1.8% to 19.6%. But, they noticed that no deaths occurred in the vaccinated men. They expressed, "We accept that the utilization of killed cultures as described prevented the improvement of the sickness in a considerable lot of our work personnel and modified its course great in others." The investigators reasoned that B. influenzae played no role in the outbreak.

E. C. Rosenow (Mayo Clinic) gave an account of the utilization of a mixed bacterial vaccine in Rochester, Minnesota, where around 21,000 people got three dosages of a vaccine in his underlying investigation. He presumed that "The total incidence of recognizable flu, pneumonia, and encephalitis in the inoculated is roughly 33% above that of the uninoculated control. The complete death rate from flu or pneumonia is only one-fourth in the inoculated as compared with the uninoculated." He would proceed to test his vaccine for almost 100,000 people.

In a publication entitled "Prophylactic Inoculation against Influenza," the Journal of the American Association of Medicine editors warned that "the information presented is just too insufficient even to consider permitting a competent judgment" of whether the vaccines were viable. Specifically, they addressed to Rosenow's paper:

"To specify just one case: The experience with a Rochester clinic—where fourteen nurses (out of what number of?)

created flu inside two days (what number of prior?) preceding the first inoculation (at what period in the plague?), and just one case (out of what number of conceivable outcomes?) grew along these lines during a time of about a month and a half—may be copied, undoubtedly, in the experience of different observers utilizing no vaccines whatever. Except if all the cards are on the table, and except if we know so far as conceivable all the elements that may impact the outcomes, we can't have a good reason for deciding if the consequences of prophylactic inoculation against flu justify the translation they have gotten in certain quarters."

ESTIMATING ACHIEVEMENT

None of the immunizations portrayed above forestalled viral flu contamination; we know because flu is brought about by an infection, and none of the antibodies secured against it. However, were any of them defensive against the bacterial diseases that created the flu? Vaccinologist Stanley A. Plotkin, MD, thinks they were most certainly not. He let us know, "The bacterial vaccines produced for Spanish flu were most likely ineffective because at the time it was not realized that pneumococcal microscopic organisms come in many, numerous serotypes and that of the bacterial gathering they called B. influenzae, is just one part of the significant pathogen." At the end of the day, the vaccine designers had little capacity to recognize, separate, and produce all the possible disease-causing strains of bacteria. Surely, the present pneumococcal vaccine for youngsters secures against 13 serotypes of that microorganisms, and the vaccine for adults protects ensures against 23 serotypes.

A 2010 article, however, describes a meta-examination of bacterial vaccine studies from 1918-19 and recommends an increasingly good understanding. In light of the 13 examinations that met inclusion criteria, the authors presume that a portion of the antibodies could have reduced the attack rate of pneumonia after a viral flu infection. They recommend that, despite the restricted quantities of microscopic organism's strains in the antibodies, inoculation could have prompted cross-protection from different related strains.

It was not until the 1930s that analysts built up that flu was in truth brought about by an infection, not a bacterium. Pfeiffer's flu bacillus would eventually be named Haemophilus influenzae, the name holding the heritage of its long-standing, but incorrect relationship with flu. And, today, flu vaccines, just as H. influenzae type b vaccines, are generally available to prevent illness.

Clinical Performances of the Day

In 1918, there was an incomplete recognition of the flu viral disease. It was believed to be a bacterial disease at that point. The study of virology was in its earliest stages, and microscopes of the era were not sufficiently able to view such minor sub-life forms. While in the years paving the way to the pandemic there were vaccines made to fight diseases like rabies and tuberculosis, the emphasis on defeating a bacterium referred to as Pfeiffer's bacillus, which was wrongly accepted to be answerable for the influenza outbreak, distracted the medical community of the time.

A nursing volunteer, Lutiant Van Wert from the Haskell Institute, depicted what steady consideration resembled in a letter home to a friend. She described the utilization of drugs (transcendently anti-inflammatory medicine), observing temperature, applying ice packs to those with high fevers, taking care of the wiped out, and applying camphorated sweet oils to their chests.

While headache medicine was the best drug for fevers around then, it was moderately new, and the dosing was far higher than what might be viewed as safe levels today. It was entirely expected to give doses in the scope of 8 to 30 grams to flu patients; by comparison, today's dosages max at 3 grams for each day in partitioned dosages. This may have exacerbated their conditions by inhibiting clotting, causing hyperventilation, and worsening edema or liquid in the lungs.

Why the 1918 Spanish influenza challenged both memory and imagination

In June 1987, a gathering of activists assembled in San Francisco to express their feelings of appreciation to friends and lovers who had recently died of AIDS. When numerous survivors of the 'gay plague,' as the infection was then alluded to in the media, were being denied strict internments, it felt essential to respect them.

To guarantee the deceased were not overlooked, Cleve Jones, a San Francisco gay activist, hit on the picture the labels of 40 AIDS fatalities on notices, hanging them from the balcony of City Hall.

Lined up beside one another, the bulletins took after nothing so much as a quilt. What wondered Jones is if he somehow managed to make a real quilt with each panel estimating the size of a normal grave? Furthermore, imagine a scenario in which the boards were laid head to toe at a national milestone. It would be an appropriate honoring, and, he contemplated, an image government officials would not be possible to overlook.

Almost in October 1987, on the event of a mass walk for lesbian and gay rights in Washington DC, the main segment of the AIDS Memorial Quilt weaved with the labels of 1,920 victims, laid on the National Mall. Today the quilt has almost 50,000 boards and weighs roughly 54 tons, making it the biggest part of network people art on the planet and, all the more significantly, the weightiest memorial to any pandemic ever.

Skulls, skeletons, and stones

Helps isn't the main pandemic to have inspired artistic productions. In the wake of the fourteenth-century Black Death, specialists finished places of worship and the tombs of victims with horrifying pictures of moving skeletons, a reference to the mania for dancing that held towns in the way of the plague bacillus.

By the sixteenth century, the recurrent European experience of plague had spurred a creative cottage industry, with portrait painters like Albrecht Dürer and Frans Hals depicting well off patrons holding skulls and other keepsakes more as tokens of their mortality.

All the more as of late, the call to honor victims of the West African Ebola pandemic has seen the assembly of a burial ground at the site of an Ebola treatment unit in Foya, Liberia, where 5,000 Liberians and health workers died in 2014. The principal thing that welcomes guests at the entranceway is a large marble stone recorded with the legend: "Those let go here will never be overlooked."

However, what if a pandemic that killed far more than AIDS and Ebola combined?

Between the spring of 1918 and the winter of 1919, the 'Spanish flu,' so called because Spain was the first country to acknowledge the spreading disease, spread over the globe, killing an estimated 50–100 million individuals. (By examination, until this point in time, 35 million have died from AIDs, and 12,000 died in the 2014–16 Ebola epidemic.)

Yet, even in this, the centennial year of the pandemic, you will find no memorials to Spanish influenza, compared with the AIDS quilt, and few graveyards memorial parks recognizing the sacrifice of doctors and nurses. Nor will you find numerous books, tunes, or gems from the period that refer to the 1918 pandemic.

The enigma of cultural amnesia

This absence of artistic responses and cognizant demonstrations of public remembrance puzzled at that point. "There is some psychological enthusiasm to the realization that the emotional impression made [by the flu pandemic] was fainter than that delivered by considerably less grave epidemiological happening," watched Major Greenwood, a classically trained researcher and disease transmission expert who aggregated the official British government report on the pandemic in his 1935 book 'Scourges and Crowd-Diseases: An Introduction to the Study of Epidemiology.'

The environmental historian Alfred Crosby was similarly confused; writing in his history of the pandemic in 1976, he stated, "One scan for clarifications for the odd actuality that Americans took little notification of the pandemic, and then quickly forgot whatever they noticed." Crosby's book was initially entitled 'Plague and Peace.' In any case, in 1989, in the wake of the AIDS pandemic, his publishers reissued the title as 'America's Forgotten Pandemic,' along these lines counterpoising the distress, stun, and frightfulness of AIDS with the cultural amnesia then surrounding the Spanish flu.

Grief behind closed doors

So what makes a few scourges and pandemics be forgotten and others to be remembered? To answer that, we have to see how this season's flu virus struck individuals at that point.

While 100m is an impressive number, those deaths were spread the world over, and on account of Britain (225,000 deaths) and the United States (675,000 deaths) spoke to only 2 percent of those countries' populations. Indeed, even in India, where the Spanish influenza is estimated to have killed 18.5m, the death rate was only 6 percent.

On the other hand, the Black Death is estimated to have killed between 30 to 60 percent of Europe's population in the central years of the fourteenth century (40–70m individuals, as Suzanna Austin calculates in 'A Pest in the Land: new world pandemics in a worldwide point of view,' distributed in 2003). When Europe's population was tremendously reduced by famine, the repeated waves of plague also had a significant segment impact, bringing about a lack of agricultural workers. This expanded the bargaining power of the peasants and, as indicated by certain history specialists, encouraged the collapse of the feudal system.

Shouldn't something be said about the deaths themselves? The last phase of the Spanish influenza was a grisly affair, with the worst-affected individuals capitulating to a condition considered as cyanosis that saw their lips, cheeks, and ears turn a purple-blue color as their lungs loaded up with choking fluids.

Yet, while the cyanosis was invariably fatal, the side effects presented in just about portion of the aspiratory cases and a large portion of the deaths happened away from public scrutiny in the security of individuals' homes. Balance this with Kaposi's sarcoma, the alarming skin condition that, combined with the visible wasting of muscle and substance, made early AIDS patients so shocking to behold.

In the early long periods of the pandemic, AIDS appeared to single out gay men and other so-called 'at-risk groups, for example, Haitians and heroin clients. As places of worship wouldn't cover victims and schools barred hemophiliacs infected with the infection through contaminated blood products, it is obvious that the shame and grief of friends immediately went to outrage and requests for political change.

By contrast, even when the Spanish flu mutated into a virulent killer in the autumn of 1918, the vast majority of the deaths were compressed into a short four-week time frame, with the mortality falling on a wide cross-area of society. Cutting across social, sexual, and ethnic lines, it didn't turn into a vehicle for stigma or a motor for outrage.

Deaths that defy imagination

But perhaps the biggest reason for the nonappearance of open dedications to the Spanish influenza is the impossibility of imagining deaths on such a scale. In his novel 'The Plague,' Albert Camus describes the huge number of bodies from the past as close to an intangible mist drifting through the mind.

In any case, in this, the centennial year of the pandemic might be evolving. To correspond with the 100th commemoration of the savage fall wave, the Florence Nightingale Museum opened another presentation in September 2018, welcoming us to recollect the wartime experiences of specialists and nurses, a considerable lot of whom sacrificed their lives thinking about flu patients.

CHAPTER 5 - BIOGRAPHICAL TESTIMONIES

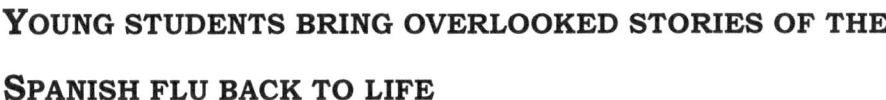

YOUNG STUDENTS BRING OVERLOOKED STORIES OF THE SPANISH FLU BACK TO LIFE

Through her school's honor winning history project on the Spanish Flu pandemic, 11-year-old Tyya Strutt took in a solemn truth.

"A great many people who died in times of terrible events or risk are always forgotten, particularly if they are youngsters," says Strutt. "But this isn't correct."

Strutt and her Grade 5/6 class, at Dundas Central Elementary School in Dundas, Ontario, explored the account of Hazel Layden, a 15-year-old who died from the Spanish Flu in 1918. The students were attracted by Layden's story since she was a student at their school (a legacy-building worked in 1857).

"It was significant when we learned that Hazel went to our school, and she even learned in our homeroom," reflects Strutt. "She sat in a similar room where we have our classes, and she played on a similar play area like us.

Hazel's story meant a great deal to us, most likely because this woman was one of us." ~ Tyya Strutt

The lecture, drove by teacher Rob Bell, won an honor for the Recovering Canada challenge. Across the country, rivalry runs in 2018-2019 that challenged Canadians to share forgotten stories of the Spanish Flu pandemic. The challenge finished in an awards ceremony that occurred at the Canada Science and Technology Museum on May 11, 2019.

"At the point when we heard that we had won the award, our initial response was feelings of shock, pride, satisfaction, and excitement," says Strutt.

The nationwide competition was prepared by "Defining Moments Canada," an online network giving digital research and storytelling tools in remembrance of the centennial of the Spanish Flu plague. A catastrophic event, the Spanish Flu affected millions; yet the accounts of Canadians implicated have gone to a great extent untold.

A deadly and largely forgotten enemy

To place the effect of the Spanish Flu pandemic into point of view, think about the First World War, which was perhaps the deadliest conflicts in worldwide history. It killed more than 9,000,000 combatants and more than 7,000,000 regular citizens as an immediate consequence of the war. The end of this contention on November 11, 1918, and the penance made by those in the line of obligation is recollected and celebrated every year all around the world. But then, 1918-1919 was spooky by an even more deadly, and to a great extent forgotten enemy: The Spanish Flu. In the only a year and a half, more than 33% of the total population was contaminated, and 50 to 100 million individuals passed on; this is more than the Black Death, and more than the First and Second World Wars consolidated.

For the centenary celebration, 'Defining Moments Canada' has driven an investigation of these stories using digital media. Here is a couple of a greater amount of the remarkable stories of Canadians who had their lives perpetually modified by the Spanish Flu pandemic.

Blanche-Olive Lavallée and the starting points of the Spanish Flu

Blanche-Olive Lavallée was a French-Canadian medical caretaker from Montréal who enrolled in the Canadian Expeditionary Force to serve in Europe. She was recruited to an emergency clinic outside of Paris, France, in May 1915. Blanche-Olive was responsible for a working room in what got one of the busiest Canadian Hospitals because of its proximity to combat zones. Her hours would have been loaded up with an endless flow of wounded, and her rest would have been constantly interrupted by the hints of mounted gun discharge. By 1917, the physical cost from exhaustion and stress was extraordinary to the point that Blanche-Olive was routinely experiencing incessant infected appendix, pallor, and general weakness.

To exacerbate the situation, in the spring of 1918, nurses and doctors began to see an extreme and especially destructive infection spreading quickly around the squeezed military sleeping enclosure. Effectively debilitated from long periods of strenuous conditions, Blanche-Olive was hospitalized with pneumonia, bronchitis, flu, and an intense infected appendix, and was sent back to Canada. She, and numerous different nurses and soldiers, unconsciously conveyed the Spanish Flu pandemic back to Canada.

Amelia Earhart and the Spanish Flu in Canada

The principal genuine cases in Canada were accounted for in pre-fall 1918, in port urban areas like Halifax and Québec, where boats were coming back from war areas conveying the wounded and ill. Despite efforts to quarantine the debilitated, the infection spread quickly. At first, patients had typical influenza-like symptoms: headaches, weakness, fevers, aches, and sore throats. But, as the illness occured, body liquid could develop, hindering circulation and filling the lungs. At last, most deaths were brought about by pneumonia, an optional disease inside the lungs.

In Toronto, the pandemic hit in September 1918. The medical clinics filled rapidly. Antiviral medications didn't exist, and within the close confines of the emergency clinics, numerous parental figures became sick. One of these attendants was Amelia Earhart, of flying acclaim, who was working at the Spadina Military Hospital on the University of Toronto grounds. She endures seasonal influenza, yet built up a severe sinus infection that took necessary medical procedure and a whole year to heal.

ELIZABETH "KIRKINA" JEFFERIES MUCKO AND THE EFFECT ON GENERAL WELLBEING

The nation over, all ages, all classes, and what not networks were susceptible. Whole families became sick. Elizabeth "Kirkina" Jefferies Mucko was an Inuit lady from Labrador. Along with her significant other Adam Mucko, she brought seven youngsters up in the Sandwich Bay region on the Labrador coast. This people group was especially hard-hit by the pandemic, losing 20 percent of the population to flu. Elizabeth's whole family became sick, and tragically, her husband and six of their children died. Since the family was quite isolated, Elizabeth needed to cover her family herself.

With no antibiotics (they hadn't been invented at this point), doctors and public health officials had restricted treatment tools. Rather, they depended on promoting preventative measures among the general population. These included: shutting open spaces like schools and theaters, guaranteeing proper ventilation in buildings, covering your mouth when hacking, isolate measures, and wearing masks. However, considering the size, public health officials were criticized for utilizing outdated and inadequate measures. This led to the formation of the government Department of Health in 1919.

Honoring memories

By correlation with the First World War, the difficult history of the Spanish Flu in Canada has been everything, but overlooked. In celebration, Defining Moments Canada assembled a portion of the overlooked accounts of people, explicit groups, and certain networks to archive their interesting encounters and respect their memory.

The learners of Dundas Central Public School never figured out how to discover an image of Hazel Layden; no school photograph was taken that year because of the Spanish Flu plague. Her memory may have blurred into a lack of definition, alongside a huge number of other people who capitulated to the pandemic. Rather, through crafting by these young students, Hazel's legacy will live on.

Survivors Remember 1918 Worldwide Flu Pandemic

At the height of this season's flu virus pandemic in 1918, William H. Sardo Jr. recollects the pine caskets stacked in the lounge room of his family's home, a burial service home in Washington, D.C.

The city had eased back to a close to end. Schools were shut. Faith gatherings were banned. The federal government limited its long stretches of activity. Individuals have died; some who became sick in the first part of the day was dead by night.

"That is the way quickly it happened," said Sardo, 94, who lives in a helped living office simply outside the country's capital. "They vanished from the essence of the earth."

Sardo is among the last overcomers of the 1918 influenza pandemic. Their accounts offer a brief look at the forgotten history of one of the world's worst plagues, when the infection killed at any rate, 50 million individuals and perhaps as many as 100 million.

More than 600,000 individuals in the United States died of what was then called "Spanish Influenza." This season's flu virus appeared to be especially deadly for, in any case, healthy young adults, a large number of whom suffocated from the buildup of liquids in their lungs.

In the United States, the principal revealed cases surfaced at an Army camp in Kansas as World War I started slowing down. The infection immediately spread among officers at U.S. camps and in the channels of Europe. It paralyzed numerous communities as it circled the world.

In the District of Columbia, the primarily recorded flu death came on Sept. 21, 1918. The person in question, a 24-year-old railroad worker, had been exposed in New York four days earlier. This flu moved through the country's capital, which had pulled in a great many troopers and war workers. When the pandemic had died down, in any event, 30,000 individuals had become sick, and 3,000 had died in the city.

Flu 'made everybody afraid.'

Among the tainted was Sardo, who was 6 years old at the time.

He remembers little of his sickness but reviews that his mom was terrified.

"They kept me all-around isolated from everyone," said Sardo, who lived with his folks, two siblings, and three other relatives. His family quarantined him in the room he had shared with his sibling. Everybody in the family wore masks.

The city started closing down. The central government staggered its hours to constrain swarming in the city and streetcars. Commissioners overseeing the region closed schools toward the beginning of October, alongside play areas, theaters, vaudeville houses, and "all spots of amusement." Dances and other get-togethers were banned.

The chiefs requested that ministry drop community gatherings because the pandemic was threatening the "tools of the federal government," The Washington Star paper detailed at that point. Ministers protested.

"There was a feeling that they couldn't go to God, other than in prayer," Sardo said. "They loved the feeling of going to chapel, and they were forbidden."

Seasonal influenza's spread and the following restrictions "made everyone hesitant to go and see anyone," he said.

"It changed a ton of society," Sardo said. "We became more individualistic."

At that point, rumors swirled that the Germans had spread the sickness — which Sardo didn't accept.

In a list of 12 principles to prevent the disease's spread, the Army's top health spokesperson wrote that individuals should "avoid needless crowding," open windows and "breathe deeply" when the air is "pure" and "wash your hands before eating."

One motto was, "Conceal each cough and sneeze. If you don't, you'll spread the sickness."

The healthy individuals wore covers while venturing outside. People who were known to be tainted were threatened with a $50 fine in case they were found out in public. Sardo remembers individuals throwing buckets of water with disinfectant on their walkways to wash away germs from individuals spitting in the city.

These days, government health officials are attempting to build their case for school closings and similar steps during a future flu pandemic by showcasing new research that proposes such measures appeared to work during the fatal Spanish flu of 1918.

Scientists found that urban areas like St. Louis, which founded "social distancing" at any rate fourteen days before flu cases peaked in their networks, had flu-related death rates not exactly a large portion of that of Philadelphia, which didn't act until some other time.

The whirlwind historical research project, which began in August and was revealed for the current month, included a group of analysts from the University of Michigan and the U.S. Communities for Disease Control and Prevention. They searched through health records, newspaper clippings and different documents from 45 cities.

Another finding: The more social distancing measures were utilized, and the more they were set up, the less extreme was the pandemic's impact on a specific city. Wearing masks in public, restricting door-to-door sales, dropping church, and isolating debilitated individuals were among the layers of measures that seemed helpful.

How the Terrible 1918 Flu Spread crossways America Haskell County, Kansas, lies in the southwest corner of the state, close to Oklahoma and Colorado. In 1918, turf houses were as yet normal, barely distinguishable from the treeless, dry prairie they were dug out of. It had been steers nation, a presently bankrupt farm, once took care of 30,000 head, but Haskell farmers also raised swine, which is one potential piece of information to the starting point of the emergency that would threaten the world that year. Another sign is that the area sits on a major migratory flyway for 17 bird species, including sand hill cranes and mallards. Researchers today understand that bird influenza viruses, like human influenza viruses, can also contaminate pigs. When a bird virus and a human infection taint a similar pig cell, their various qualities can be rearranged and traded like playing a game of cards, bringing about another, maybe particularly deadly, infection.

We can't state for sure what occurred in 1918 in Haskell County; however, we do realize that a flu outbreak struck in January; an outbreak so severe that, although flu was not then a "reportable" sickness, a local physician named Loring Miner, a large and forceful man, abrupt, and a player in local political issues, who turned into a specialist before the acknowledgment of the germ hypothesis of malady, but whose scholarly interest had kept him side by the side of logical turns of events, went to the difficulty of alarming the U.S. General Health Service. The report itself does not exist anymore, yet it remains as the primarily recorded notification anyplace in the realm of surprising flu movement that year. The neighborhood paper, the Santa Fe Monitor, affirms that something odd was going on around that time: "Mrs. Eva Van Alstine is wiped out with pneumonia, Ralph Lindeman is still very sick.., Homer Moody has been accounted for very sick, Pete Hesser's three youngsters have pneumonia, Mrs. J.S. Cox is frail, yet Ralph McConnell has been very debilitated this week. Mertin, the youthful child of Ernest Elliot, is wiped out with pneumonia. Almost everyone over the country has lagniappe or pneumonia."

A few Haskell men who had been presented with the flu went camping in Funston, central Kansas. Days after the fact, on March 4, the first soldier known to have flu was detailed sick. The enormous Army base was preparing men for battle in World War I, and inside about fourteen days, 1,100 soldiers were admitted to the hospital, with thousands of the more sick in barracks. Thirty-eight kicked the bucket. At that point, infected troopers likely carried flu from Funston to other Army camps in the States; 24 of 36 huge camps had outbreaks, sickening many thousands, and preceding carrying the illness abroad.

The flu infection transforms quickly, changing enough that the human safe framework experiences issues recognizing and attacking it, even starting with one season, then into the next. A pandemic happens when a completely new and destructive flu infection, which the immune framework has not recently been observed, enters the population and spreads around the world.

Common occasional flu infections typically tie just to cells in the upper respiratory tract, the nose and throat, which is the reason they transmit without any problem. The 1918 pandemic infection contaminated cells in the upper respiratory tract, transmitting effectively, but also deep into the lungs, harming tissue and regularly prompting viral, as well as bacterial pneumonia.

Although a few scientists contend that the 1918 pandemic started somewhere else in France in 1916 or China and Vietnam in 1917, numerous different investigations demonstrated a U.S. root. Through the vast majority of career studying influenza, the end proof was "strongly suggestive" that the sickness began in the United States and spread to France with "the appearance of American troops." Camp Funston had, for quite some time, been considered as the site where the pandemic began until my historical research, published in 2004, highlighted an earlier outbreak in Haskell County.

In any place it started, the pandemic lasted only 15 months, yet was the deadliest disease outbreak in humanity's history, killing between 50 million and 100 million individuals around the world, as indicated by the most broadly referred to investigation. A careful worldwide number is unlikely ever to be resolved, given the absence of appropriate records in a significant part of the world around then. But the pandemic killed a larger number of individuals in a year than AIDS has executed in 40 years, and more than the bubonic plague slaughtered in a century.

The effect of the pandemic on the United States is sobering to consider: Some 670,000 Americans died.

In 1918, medication had barely gotten to present day level; a few researchers, despite everything accepted, "miasma" accounted for flu's spread. With medication advances from that point forward, laypeople have gotten somewhat self-satisfied about flu. Today we stress over Ebola or Zika or MERS or other colorful pathogens, and not over a disease regularly confused for the basic virus. This is a mistake.

We are arguably as powerless or more vulnerable to another pandemic as we were in 1918. Today top public health experts routinely rank flu as conceivably the most dangerous "emerging" health risk we face. Prior to this year, after leaving his post as leader of the Centers for Disease Control and Prevention, Tom Frieden was asked what terrified him the most, and what kept him up around evening time. "The greatest concern is consistently for a flu pandemic. It's truly the worst-case scenario." So the awful occasions of 100 years prior have a surprising urgency, particularly since the most crucial exercises to be gained from the disaster have not yet been absorbed.

At first, the 1918 pandemic set off not many alarms, primarily because in many spots, it once in a while killed, despite the huge quantities of individuals infected. Specialists in the British Grand Fleet, for instance, conceded 10,313 soldiers wiped out straight in May and June, but just 4 died.

It had hit both warring armed forces in France in April, yet troops excused it as "three-day fever." The main consideration it got came when it traveled through Spain, and sickened the ruler; the press in Spain, which was not at war, composed finally on the disease, in contrast to the blue-penciled press in warring countries, including the United States. Consequently, it got known as "Spanish influenza." By June, flu came from Algeria to New Zealand. A recent report finished up, "In numerous parts of the world, the primary wave either was such a blackout as to be hardly perceptible or was by and large lacking, and was wherever of a mild form." Some specialist's argued that it was too gentle to even think about being flu.

However, there were warnings, ominous ones. Although a couple passed on in the spring, the individuals who did were regularly healthy young adults, individuals whom flu once rarely kill. To a great extent, local outbreaks were not all that gentle. A single French Army post of 1,018 officers, 688 were hospitalized, and 49 died; five percent of that population of young men, dead. And, a few deaths in the primary wave were neglected because they were misdiagnosed regularly as meningitis. A puzzled Chicago pathologist watched lung tissue heavy with liquid and "full of hemorrhages" and asked as to whether it spoke to "a new disease."

The medical clinic at Camp Devens, an Army training base 35 miles from Boston that teemed with 45,000 officers, could suit 1,200 patients. On September 1, it held 84.

On September 7, a fighter sent to the hospital, delirious and screaming, when examined was diagnosed to have meningitis. The following day twelve additional men from his organization were diagnosed to have meningitis. But, as more men became sick, doctors changed the finding to flu. Out of nowhere, an Army report noticed, "Influenza...occurred as an explosion."

At the outbreak's peak, 1,543 soldiers detailed sick with flu in a single day. Presently, with hospitals facilities overwhelmed, with doctors and nurses sick, and with too not many cafeteria workers to take care of patients and staff, the hospital ceased accepting patients, regardless of how sick, leaving thousands sicker and dying in barracks.

Roy Grist, a doctor at the emergency clinic, wrote an associate, "These men start with what gives off an impression of being a common attack of LaGrippe or Influenza, and when brought to the Hosp., they quickly build up the most vicious kind of Pneumonia that has ever been seen. Two hours after confirmation they have the Mahogany spots over the cheek bones, and a couple of hours after the fact, you can start to see the Cyanosis; "the term refers to an individual diverting blue from lack of oxygen," reaching out from their ears and spreading everywhere throughout the face. It is just a matter of a couple of hours later that the very end comes. It is horrible. We have been averaging around 100 deaths for each day. For a few days, there were no final resting places, and the bodies piled up something fierce."

Devens, and the Boston region, was the first place in the Americas hit by the pandemic's subsequent wave. Before it ended, flu was all over the place, from ice-bound Alaska to steaming Africa. And, this time, it was deadly.

The killing made its horrors. Governments aggravated them, halfway on account of the war. For example, the U.S. military generally took 50% of all doctors under 45, and the greater part of the best ones.

What demonstrated considerably more deadly was the government policy towards reality. At the point when the United States entered the war, Woodrow Wilson requested that "the soul of merciless brutality enter into the very fiber of national life." So he made the Committee on Public Information, which was roused by a guide who expressed, "Truth and lie are subjective terms. The power of thought lies in its moving worth. It makes almost no difference if it is true or false."

At Wilson's asking, Congress passed the Sedition Act, making it culpable with 20 years in jail to "absolute, print, write or publish any disloyal, profane, foul, or abusive language about the type of administration of the US or to ask, incite, or advocate any curtailment of creation in this country of anything or things necessary or basic to the prosecution of the war." Government banners and advertisements urged people to answer to the Justice Department anybody "who spreads pessimistic stories, cries for harmony, or belittles our push to win the war."

Against this background, while flu seeped into American life, public health officials, resolved to keep morale up, started to lie.

Right off the bat in September, a Navy transport from Boston carried flu to Philadelphia, where the disease erupted in the Navy Yard. The city's public health director, Wilmer Krusen, pronounced that he would "keep this disease to its current limits, and in this, we make certain to be effective. No fatalities have been recorded. No worry, whatever is felt."

The following day two sailors died of flu. Krusen expressed they died of "old-fashioned flu or held," not Spanish influenza. Another health official declared, "Starting now and into the foreseeable future, the disease will decrease."

The following day 14 sailors died, as well as the first civilian. Every day the disease accelerated. Everyday papers guaranteed readers that flu represented no danger. Krusen assured the city he would "stop the epidemic from really developing."

By September 26, flu had spread across the country. Thus numerous military training camps were starting to look like Devens that the Army dropped; it's across the nation draft call.

Philadelphia had scheduled a major Liberty Loan march for September 28. Specialists asked Krusen to cancel it, fearful that several thousand jamming the route, smashing against one another for a superior view, would spread malady. They persuaded columnists to compose tales about the threat. In any case, editors wouldn't run them, and would not print letters from specialists. The biggest motorcade in Philadelphia's history continued on time.

The development time of the flu is a few days. Two days after the motorcade, Krusen yielded that the scourge "now present in the civilian population was...assuming the sort found in" Army camps. He advised not to be "hysterical over misrepresented reports."

He needn't have stressed over distortion; the papers were his ally. "Logical Nursing Halting Epidemic," an Inquirer headline blared. In truth, nurses did were not affected since none were available: Out of 3,100 critical requests for nurses submitted to one dispatcher, just 193 were given. Krusen at long last and belatedly, requested all schools closed and banned every single open social occasion, yet a paper nonsensically said the request was not "a public health measure" and "there is no reason for panic or alarm."

There was a lot of cause. Even under the least favorable conditions, the scourge in Philadelphia would kill 759 people in one day. Ministers drove horse-drawn trucks down city lanes, calling upon residents to draw out their dead; many were buried in mass graves. More than 12,000 Philadelphians died—about every one of them in six weeks.

Across the country, public officials were lying. U.S. Top health spokesperson Rupert Blue stated, "There is no reason to worry if safety measures are watched." New York City's general wellbeing executive proclaimed "other bronchial infections and not the purported Spanish influenza... [Caused] the disease of most of the people who were reported for sick with flu." The Los Angeles community health chief said, "If conventional precautions are seen, there is no reason to get excited."

For a case of the press' failure, think about Arkansas. Over four days in October, the medical clinic at Camp Pike admitted 8,000 soldiers. Francis Blake, an individual from the Army's exceptional pneumonia unit, described the scene: "Every corridor and there are miles of them with double columns of bunks ...with flu patients...There is just passing and devastation." Yet seven miles far away in Little Rock, a feature in the Gazette imagined yawns: "Spanish flu is plain la grippe regular old fever and chills."

Individuals realized this was not old news, however. They knew because the numbers were staggering; in San Antonio, 53 percent of the population became ill with flu. They knew because victims could die within hours of the principal symptoms; horrific symptoms, hurts, and cyanosis, as well as frothy blood, hacked up from the lungs and seeping from the nose, ears, and even eyes. Also, individuals knew because towns and cities ran out of coffins.

Individuals could think nothing they were being told, so they feared everything, especially the unknown. To what extent would it last? What number of, would it murder? Who might it murder? With reality covered, morale collapsed. Society itself started to deteriorate.

In many disasters, people meet up, help one another, as we saw as of late with Hurricanes Harvey and Irma. But in 1918, without leadership, and without reality, trust evaporated. And people took care of just themselves.

In Philadelphia, the head of Emergency Aid argued, "All who are liberated from the care of the sick at home report as ahead of schedule as possible on emergency work." But volunteers didn't come. The Bureau of Child Hygiene asked individuals to take in just temporarily, children whose parents were dying or dead; few answered. Crisis Aid again argued, "We just should have more volunteer helpers. These individuals are practically all at the point of death. Won't you come to our assistance?" Still nothing.

At last, Emergency Aid's director turned bitter and contemptuous: "Many women had wonderful dreams of themselves in the roles of angels of mercy. Nothing appears to rouse them now. There are families in which the kids are starving because there is nobody to give them food. The death rate is so high that they, despite everything, calm down."

Philadelphia's misery was not exceptional. A couple and three youngsters were all sick together, at the same time; a Red Cross specialist detailed, "Not one of the neighbors would come in and help. I called the lady's sister. She came and tapped on the window, but wouldn't converse with me until she had gotten a protected separation away." In New Haven, Connecticut, John Delano reviewed, "Regularly when somebody was wiped out in those days, people would bring food over from different families, but nobody was coming in, and no one would get food, no one dropped by." In Perry County, Kentucky, the Red Cross section director asked for help, and argued that there were "many cases of individuals starving to death, not from lack of food but since the well was hysterical and would not go close to the wiped out."

In Goldsboro, North Carolina, Dan Tonkel reviewed, "We were very afraid to breathe. You were afraid even to go out. The fear was so extraordinary that individuals were afraid to leave their homes, and afraid to talk with each other." In Washington, D.C., William Sardo stated, "It kept individuals separately. You had no college life, you had no congregation life, you had nothing. It destroyed all family and network life. The terrifying angle was the point at which every day unfolded you didn't know whether you would be there when the sun set that day."

An interior American Red Cross report concluded that, "A fear and panic of the flu, much the same as the fear of the Middle Ages concerning the Black Plague, [has] been prevalent in numerous parts of the country."

Fear emptied places of employment, and emptied cities. Shipbuilding workers all through the Northeast were advised they were as essential to the war exertion, as officers at the front. However, at the L.H. Shattuck Co., just 54 percent of its workers appeared; at the George A. Gilchrist yard, just 45 percent did; at Freeport Shipbuilding just 43 percent; at Groton Iron Works, 41 percent.

Fear emptied the streets, as well. A clinical student working in a crisis medical clinic in Philadelphia, one of the nation's largest cities, experienced not many vehicles out, and he took to counting them. One night, traveling the 12 miles home, he saw not a single car. "The life of the city had nearly stopped," he said.

On the opposite side of the globe, in Wellington, New Zealand, another man stepped outside his crisis medical clinic and found something very similar: "I remained in Wellington City at 2 P.M. on a weekday evening, and there was not a spirit to be seen; no cable cars are running; no shops open, and the main traffic was a van with a white sheet attached to the side with a major red cross painted on it, filling in as an emergency vehicle or funeral car. It was a city of the dead."

Victor Vaughan, once in the past, the dean of the University of Michigan's Medical School, was not a man to resort to hyperbole. Presently the leader of the Army's infectious disease division, he jotted down his private fear: "If the scourge proceeds with its mathematical rate of acceleration, civilization could easily disappear from the substance of the earth inside a matter of a couple of more weeks."

At that point, as out of nowhere as it came, the flu appeared to disappear. It had consumed the available fuel in a given network. An inclination of unease remained; however, helped by the happiness going with the end of the war, traffic came back to streets, schools and organizations reopened, and society returned to normal.

A third wave followed in January 1919, finishing off with the spring. This was deadly by any standard aside from the second wave, and one specific case would excellently effect on history.

On April 3, 1919, during the Versailles Peace Conference, Woodrow Wilson fell. His unexpected shortcoming and extreme confusion halfway through that gathering, broadly remarked upon, perhaps added to his abandoning his principles. The outcome was the disastrous peace treaty, which would later add to the beginning of World War II. A few students of history have attributed Wilson's confusion to a minor stroke. He had a 103-degree temperature, extreme coughing fits, diarrhea, and different genuine symptoms. A stroke explains none of the symptoms. Flu, which was then boundless in Paris and killed a young aide to Wilson, clarifies every one of them, including his confusion. Experts would later concur that numerous patients afflicted by the pandemic flu had cognitive or psychological symptoms. As a legitimate 1927 clinical review concluded, "There is no doubt that the neuropsychiatric impacts of flu are profound, and is hardly second to its impact on the respiratory system."

After that third wave, the 1918 virus didn't leave; however, it lost its extraordinary lethality, partly because numerous human safe systems currently remembered it, and halfway because it lost the capacity to invade the lungs easily. Not, at this point, a bloodthirsty murderer, it advanced into the seasonal flu.

Researchers and different specialist areas are still asking questions about the virus and the devastation it caused, including why the subsequent wave was a great deal more lethal than the first. Analysts aren't sure, and some contend that the main wave was brought about by a standard occasional flu infection that was unique about the pandemic virus. Yet, the proof appears to be overpowering that the pandemic virus had both a mild and virulent form, causing gentle. just as severe spring outbreaks, and then, for reasons that stay unclear, the harmful type of the virus turned out to be more common in the fall.

Another question concerns who died. Although the loss of life was historic, a great many people who were infected by the pandemic infection virus survived; in the developed world, the general mortality was around 2 percent. In the less evolved world, mortality was more awful. In Mexico, appraisals of the dead range from 2.3 to 4 percent of the whole population. Quite a bit of Russia and Iran saw 7 percent of the populace bite the dust. In the Fiji Islands 14 percent of the inhabitants passed on in 16 days. A 33% of the number of inhabitants in Labrador died. In little local towns in Alaska and Gambia, everybody died, likely because all became ill all the while and nobody could give care, or give individuals water, and maybe because, with such a great amount of death around them, the individuals who may have to endure didn't battle.

The age of the casualties was likewise striking. Ordinarily, old individuals represent the overwhelming number of flu deaths; in 1918, that was switched, with young adults killed in the most noteworthy numbers. This impact was elevated inside specific subgroups. For example, a

Metropolitan Life Insurance Company study of people aged 25 to 45 found that 3.26 percent of every single industrial worker and 6 percent of all coal miners died. Other studies found that for pregnant ladies, casualty rates went from 23 percent to 71 percent.

For what reason did such a large number of young adults die? As it occurs, youthful adults have the strongest immune systems, which attacked the virus with all weapons possible, including synthetic concoctions called cytokines and other microbe-fighting toxins, and the front line was the lung. These "cytokine storms" further harmed the patient's tissue. The decimation, as per the prominent flu master Edwin Kilbourne, looked like nothing to such an extent as the injuries from breathing toxic poison gas.

Occasional flu is bad enough. In current times, it killed 3,000 to 48,000 Americans every year, contingent upon the predominant virus strains available for use, in addition to other things. Furthermore, more deadly possibilities loom.

Lately, two different bird influenza viruses have been tainting individuals directly: the H5N1 strain has struck in numerous countries, while H7N9 is as yet limited to China (see "The Birth of a Killer"). By and large, these two avian flu viruses had killed 1,032 out of the 2,439 individuals infected as of this past July, a shocking death rate. Researchers state that both infection strains, up until this point, tie just to cells somewhere down in the lung and don't go from person to person. If it is possible that one obtains the capacity to contaminate the upper respiratory tract, through mutation or by swapping genes with current human infection, a fatal pandemic is possible.

Provoked by the reappearance of avian flu, governments, NGOs, and significant organizations around the globe have poured resources into getting ready for a pandemic. Due to my history of the 1918 pandemic, The Great Influenza, I was asked to partake in some from those efforts.

Public health experts agree that the most elevated need is to build up a "universal vaccine" that presents immunity against virtually all flu infections liable to infect people (see "How to Stop a Lethal Virus"). Without such a vaccine, if another pandemic infection surfaces, we should create an antibody explicitly for it; doing so will take periods and the immunization may offer just minor insurance.

Another key advance to improving pandemic status is to expand research on antiviral drugs; none is exceptionally successful against flu, and a few strains have gained protection from the antiviral drug Tamiflu.

At that point, there are less exciting measures, known as no pharmaceutical interventions: hand-washing, working from home, covering coughs, staying home when wiped out as opposed to going to work, and, if the pandemic is severe enough, boundless school closings and possibly more extreme controls. The expectation is that "layering" such activities one on another will decrease the effect of an epidemic on public health and assets in the present and in the nick of time economy. In any case, the adequacy of such interventions will rely upon open consistency, and the open should believe what it is being told.

That is the reason, in my view, the most significant exercise from 1918 is to come clean. Although that thought is consolidated into each readiness plan I am aware of, and its actual implementation will rely upon the character and leadership of the individuals in control when a crisis erupts.

I took an interest in a pandemic "war game" in Los Angeles involving area public health officials. Before the activity started, I gave a discussion about what occurred in 1918, how society separated and emphasized that to hold the public's trust, specialists must be sincere. "You don't deal with reality," I said. "You come clean." Everyone shook their heads in agreement.

Next, the individuals running the game revealed the day's test to the participants: A serious pandemic flu infection was spreading far and wide. It had not formally arrived at California, but a suspected case, and the seriousness of the indications caused it to appear to be so, had recently surfaced in Los Angeles. The news media had been educated about it and were requesting a press conference.

CHAPTER 6 - WHAT WE CAN LEARN

———— ◆ ◇ ◆ ————

EXERCISES COULD HELP AVOID A REPEAT OF ANOTHER SPANISH INFLUENZA

A pandemic ravaged the world out of control, executing more than 50 million individuals globally and around 675,000 in the US.

"The power and speed with which it struck were practically unimaginable, infecting 33% of the Earth's populace," the World Health Organization said.

That was the 1918 flu pandemic. The infection was frequently called the "Spanish influenza," although it didn't start in Spain.

Quick forward to 2020, and the novel, the current pandemic is also spreading with astonishing speed.

A portion of the painful lessons learned from the 1918 pandemic is as yet applicable today, and could help prevent a similarly catastrophic outcome.

Exercise #1: Don't ease up on social separating too early

During the Spanish influenza pandemic, individuals quit separating too soon, prompting a second wave of diseases that was deadlier than the first disease epidemiologists say.

One enormous assembling close to the end of the first wave in 1918, helped fuel the deadlier second wave.

In San Francisco, when the number of Spanish influenza cases was practically down to zero, "the city fathers stated, 'we should open up the city. How about we have a great big parade downtown. We'll all remove our masks together,'" disease transmission specialist Dr. Larry Brilliant said.

"After two months, in light of that occasion, the great flu returned thundering."

On the opposite side of the US, Philadelphia endured a similar fate.

Although 600 mariners from the Philadelphia Navy Yard had Spanish influenza in September 1918, the city didn't drop a procession booked for September 28, 1918.

After three days, Philadelphia had 635 new instances of Spanish influenza, as per the University of Pennsylvania Archives and Records Center.

"Rapidly, Philadelphia turned into the city with the highest influenza death toll in the US," Penn investigation states.

On the other hand, St. Louis, which scheduled a similar parade but dropped it fared much better.

"The following month, more than 10,000 individuals in Philadelphia died from pandemic influenza, while the loss of life in Saint Louis did not rise above 700," the US Centers for Disease Control and Prevention said.

Better places will arrive at various peaks at various occasions. But just because one spot moves past a so-called peak with coronavirus doesn't mean cases or deaths there can't rise again.

"From the picture that we have of this epidemic curve, we state that we're going to arrive at a 'peak;' we take a looks at it, and it would appear that Mt. Fuji in our brains, is a singular mountain," Brilliant said.

"I don't believe it will resemble that. I think a superior picture is a flood of a wave of a tsunami, with resonance waves that follow. Also, it's up to us how huge those different waves will be."

Exercise #2: Young, healthy adults, can be victims of their solid immune systems

The 1918 pandemic killed many young adults who were, in any case, solid, said John M. Barry, a teacher at the Tulane University School of Public Health and Tropical Medicine.

Around 66% of the deaths at that point were among individual's ages 18 to 50, "and the peak age for death was 28," said Barry, author of "The Great Influenza: The Story of the Deadliest Pandemic ever."

In the years driving up the 1918 influenza pandemic, the lifespan in the US was in the mid-50s. But, in only one year after it struck, the normal US lifespan dropped by 12 years.

Starting in 2017, the normal US lifespan was 78.6 years. Furthermore, with a current pandemic, the older and those with hidden medical issues are at higher risk for serious complications.

One explanation the 1918 influenza was so deadly for young adults was because the episode began during World War I when numerous troopers were in the military enclosure, and had closeness with one another.

"The US military preparing camps had high mortality," Barry said.

There's no world war now, yet significant exercises stay: Young, sound individuals are not strong. Also, their strong immune systems may neutralize them.

Taking a look back at Spanish influenza, researchers presently accept an "immune system overreaction added to high death rates among in any case, healthy young adults in 1918," composed Dr. Richard Gunderman, chancellor's teacher of medication at Indiana University.

A century after that pandemic, hyperactive safe frameworks could also be contributing to youngsters' deaths from a current pandemic, CNN Chief Medical Correspondent Dr. Sanjay Gupta said. These overly strong responses are regularly called cytokine storms.

"In some youthful, sound individuals, a very reactive immune system could prompt a massive inflammatory storm that could overwhelm the lungs and various organs," Gupta said.

"In those cases, it's anything but an aged or weakened immune system that is the issue; it is one that works exorbitantly well."

Exercise #3: Don't toss doubtful drugs at the virus

Indeed, there have been significant clinical and mechanical advances in the previous 102 years. But the Spanish flu and the novel coronavirus pandemics share two significant difficulties: the absence of an antibody and the lack of a fix.

In 1918, cures "changed from the recently evolved medications to oils and herbs," as indicated by a Stanford University examination into the post. "The treatment was significantly less logical than the diagnostics, as the medications had no way, from hypothesis of activity."

In 2020, there is a far reaching theory about whether hydroxychloroquine, a drug used to treat malaria, lupus, and rheumatoid joint arthritis could help current pandemic patients.

President Donald Trump has touted hydroxychloroquine, saying, "What do you need to lose? Take it." After that, some begun storing the drug although it's despite everything being tried and probably won't neutralize coronavirus.

An ongoing report discovered hydroxychloroquine didn't help hospitalized coronavirus patients - rather, a few patients created irregular heart rhythms.

"Surprisingly, and more fearful, there were responses brought about by the medication, with heart poison levels than expected; consequently, it was suspended."

Specialists in Brazil and Sweden have also raised concerns about utilizing chloroquine, a medication fundamentally the same as hydroxychloroquine, on coronavirus patients as a result of heart issues.

Exercise # 4: Social separating works

In 1918, as in 2020, travel quickly spread the infection, with U.S. soldiers making a trip toward the East Coast, on to European front lines, and carrying infection with them.

"The explanation as to why it was so savage and passed so quickly over the whole world was that it occurred during wartime," Kent says. "That is much the same as this moment of enormous globalization we are living in now."

Without the advantage of the present high-tech microscopes and genetic sequencing, specialists wrongly expected it was bacterial, and endeavors to treat it or immunize against it, fizzled with no different apparatuses to depend on, towns at last shut schools, theaters, and libraries. The National Hockey League canceled the Stanley Cup. Military leaders isolated soldiers, and community workers were encouraged to wear masks.

On the whole, 675,000 people died in the United States, more than passed on in World War II. In any case, it could have been more.

"The best way to forestall its spread was to isolate individuals from each other. A few networks did that and fared well. Others didn't and suffered high death rates," says Kent. "That exercise for us presently is significant. In case we don't gain from it, shame on us."

Exercise # 5: Viruses don't get extra for the youthful

The flu pandemic of 1918 was well on the way to hit the youthful and sound, felling individuals ages 15 to 45 with quick lethality.

"They became ill so quickly; some dropped in the avenues." Kent noticed that their appearances regularly turned pale blue red because of lack of oxygen.

As it turned out, the patients' own powerful safe systems were a piece of the issue, releasing a downpour of infection battling particles considered as cytokines that latched on to lung tissue causing lethal damage.

While the socioeconomics of current pandemic is altogether different, it's hitting more established populaces, and the resistance traded off the hardest; its behavior in the youthful and healthy is very like that of the virus a century ago. Current news reports point to immune responses called "cytokine storms" as a probable reason for the collateral damage happening in more youthful patients.

"The very same thing happened in 1918," Kent notes. "Strong immune systems overpowered different organs of the body, particularly the lungs."

Exercise # 6: Inoculation works

During the smallpox scourge that cleared across North America from 1775 to 1782, Revolutionary War soldiers took an abnormal strategy to protect themselves from the infection known as Variola major. In a procedure known as variolation (a.k.a. vaccination), they took infection stacked material from a contaminated individual's smallpox pustule, cut an entry point into the tissue of a sound patch, and focused on it.

Beneficiaries of variolation invariably got the sickness, so they were isolated. About 5% passed on. In any case, most got a mellow form of the smallpox infection.

"There is no doubt that it worked," says Fenn. "Accepting you survived it, you would gather resistance and approach the world without worrying about smallpox."

A long time later, in 1796, Edward Jenner, who himself had been variegated as a youngster, would try a similar method, taking injury material from a lady who had cowpox and rubbing it into the injury of an 8-year-old kid. At the point when he later tried to infect the kid with smallpox, no disease developed.

The idea of vaccination—named after the Latin word for cow, or Vacca, was born.

Exercise # 7: Don't blame the sick

With the spread of the current pandemic has come to a flood of hostility to Asian reaction in urban areas over the globe, driven to some degree by the way that the disease developed in the Chinese city of Wuhan and moved through the Chinese population first.

That is the same old thing, says Fenn.

"We are exceptionally inclined to blaming the individuals who become ill," she says. "It's occurred over and over throughout history."

During the cholera pandemics that hit from the 1830s to 1860s, white Protestants avoided Irish immigrants as vectors of the scourge. During the 1950s, as polio cleared the country, African Americans and the poor were focused on. During the 1980s, the fault was put on the LGBTQ people group for spreading HIV-AIDS.

"While individuals dithered around blaming (HIV-AIDS) on gay ways of life or dance club moving, valuable long periods of searching for pathogens were lost," Fenn says.

In contrast, Fenn noticed, the World Health Organization in 1980 declared that smallpox was officially the first human infectious sickness to be killed.

How was that possible? Through collaboration.

"Today, we can learn and follow up on the way that worldwide participation and sharing of information will assist us with managing these outbreaks, or we can close ourselves away and insist on going alone," says Kent.

Exercise # 8: This can end

As horrific as a current pandemic in 2020 seems to be, Kent doesn't accept its loss of life will arrive at the meteoric levels of this flu epidemic of 1918. Our general health systems, scientific tools, and clinical supplies (but hard to find) are better.

In comparison with past pandemics, we also have a head start in handling this one, concludes Fenn.

"This is the principal pandemic of this extension, where we have realized what the pathogen is from the very beginning."

The coming months willcertainly be difficult, but with social distancing set up, group resistance building, and collective work in progress to develop treatments and a vaccine, Fenn and Kent are confident.

CONCLUSION

——— ♦◇♦ ———

History reminds us that it's not the first occasion when we've survived a pandemic, and it tends to be instructive to look to the past for direction.

Past pandemics; for example, the Spanish influenza of 1918, produced strikingly similar shades of panic, political advantage, prejudice, xenophobia, and discussions around health versus the economy. Severe outbreaks also could represent the moment of truth for political pioneers. She said successful government officials didn't deny or delay. They passed on exact, timely data. There were three successive waves: the first in the spring of 1918, the second and generally deadly, was liable for 90% of deaths in the harvest time of 1918, and the last upsurge from the winter of 1918 to the spring of 1919. Before the end of the pandemic, the greater part of the total population had been infected. Estimations on mortality, and testing to confirm for lack of information have consistently been revised upwards. These days, students of history and disease transmission specialists estimate by utilizing a wide range, extending from 2.5 to

5% of the total population, which means somewhere in the range of 50 and 100 million deaths. The pandemic was, this way, five to multiple times deadlier than the First World War.

The 1918 pandemic was worldwide, with shared human catastrophe. Its outcomes were political, social, economic, and emotional. The legacy of this season's cold virus is significant: the flu infections of 1957, 1968, and 2009 are, for the most part, relatives of the H1N1 infection that caused the 1918 pandemic. The 'Spanish Flu' is an account of failure, and an image of bombed board of a pandemic for the sake of military interests.

History never repeats itself. Every chronicled second is clear from that past. By and by, relationship can be drawn between various chronicled occasions; although history doesn't show us what to do, it can rouse us to act. Looking at the 1918 flu pandemic is a chance to think about the current pandemic emergency from a different perspective.

By and by, as reviewed by Daniel Flecknoe, not the totality of the lessons have been realized: 'The way that the danger of another worldwide pandemic emerging from any modern war zone seems to once in a while highlight the political dynamic, which decides if countries do battle, and in any case shows that the exercises of 1918 have not all been very much learned. Wars debilitate the capacity of the country to prevent, detect, or fight outbreaks of infectious disease, and leave the civilian population especially vulnerable'. The outbreak of the current pandemic didn't start in a country at war. Yet, its effect is deplorable in any place where there are armed conflicts or different circumstances of violence. This difference must summon idealism. Humanity, as of now, has and will keep on finding new and powerful solution, intended to mitigate the present pandemic. In any case, for all the current logical measures to be compelling, they should be tried and subsequently understood and accepted. Trust towards specialists, public health institutions, medical researchers, and practitioners, is by and by, a key idea in times of crisis.

www.ingramcontent.com/pod-product-compliance
Lightning Source LLC
Chambersburg PA
CBHW070908080526
44589CB00013B/1227